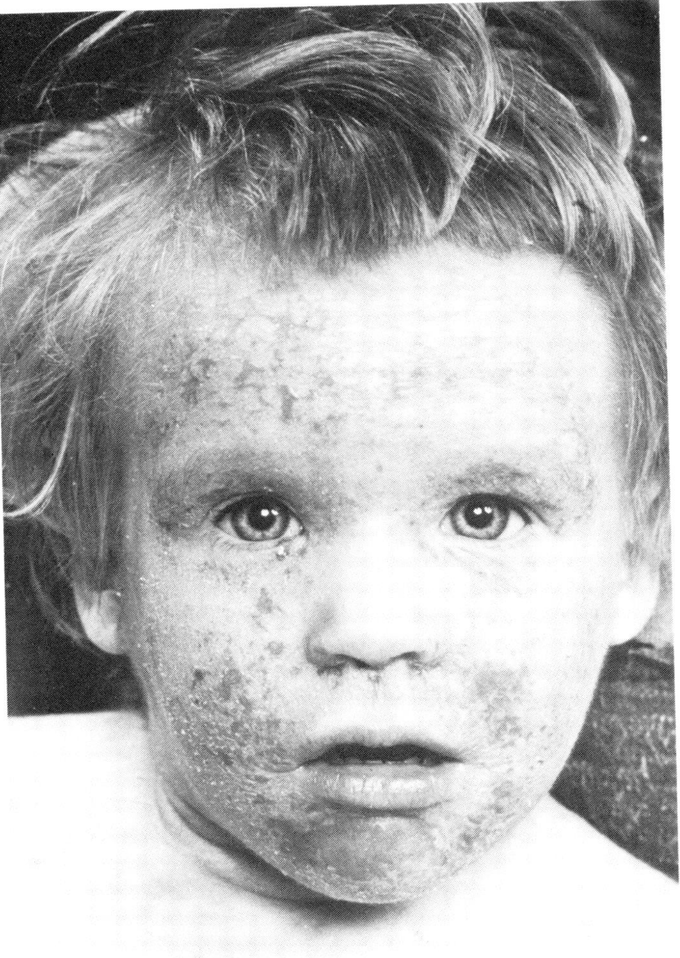

Your Child with ECZEMA

A guide for parents

Dr. David J. Atherton
MA, MB, MRCP
Consultant Dermatologist,
The Hospital for Sick Children,
Great Ormond Street,
London

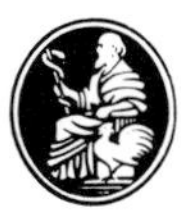

William Heinemann Medical Books Ltd
London

First published in 1984 by William Heinemann
Medical Books Ltd., 23 Bedford Square, London,
WC1B 3HH

Reprinted 1985

ISBN 0–433–00940–3

Phototypeset by Inforum Ltd, Portsmouth and
printed in Great Britain by
Redwood Burn Ltd, Trowbridge

Contents

Preface

Childhood eczema is unfortunately very common. Although it is generally a relatively minor problem, some children endure prolonged and almost unbearable suffering. The pain caused by this disease to sufferers and to their close relatives is little appreciated, and the level of help available to both groups of people leaves much to be desired. In the course of my work as a paediatric dermatologist I see many hundreds of eczematous children and their parents each year. This book has been written to provide information about the disease to parents who have a child with eczema to care for, in the hope that this will make their lives a little easier.

Parents often complain to me about their experiences with other doctors, and maybe they complain about me in the same way. Doctors are at their happiest when dealing with diseases that respond predictably and dramatically to treatment, and this is understandable. Unfortunately, severe childhood eczema is not one of these diseases and some parents feel that doctors have abandoned them to the disease. Parents often say that they have been told that nothing can be done for eczema. Sometimes I wonder whether this really is what they have been told, because nothing could be further from the truth. There is always something that can be done, and all good doctors know this. Looking after children with severe eczema can be very difficult, demanding and frustrating for a doctor, but it can also be rewarding for the same reasons. By understanding the disease better, I hope the reader will also see the doctor's problem more clearly, what he can do and what he cannot. I also hope that this will help parents and doctors to work together as a team in caring for children with eczema.

No doctor, however much he would like, has the time to cover with you more than a fraction of what is in this little book. It contains a mixture of facts, half-facts and hypotheses, and I have tried to distinguish these as far as possible. Inevitably what I have written reflects a personal view of atopic eczema, and other experts will not agree with me on every point. This is unavoidable, of course, and I make no apology for it, but it is something you should bear in mind both while reading it and when you subsequently see your child's own doctor. He may not see eczema exactly as I do, and he may be right. The key note is optimism; optimism because childhood eczema almost always fades away leaving little or no trace either physical or psychological, and optimism because research is bringing us closer to understanding the nature of this disease with the promise that, in the not too distant future, it may be prevented altogether.

I sincerely hope that you find something worth while in this book. If you do, not one of those Sunday mornings spent at my desk will have been wasted.

1 The Normal Skin

Before considering any of its diseases, it would be wrong not to take a brief look at skin in its normal state, the way it is made and the way it works. The skin has two main components, the 'epidermis' and the 'dermis', and these two together make it by far the largest organ in the body. Its function is principally to provide a barrier between our vulnerable body contents and the hostile environment outside. The importance of this function is highlighted by the fact that destruction of just 30% of a child's skin by burning is frequently fatal, whatever treatment is undertaken. There are two major components to this barrier function. One is the prevention of water loss from the body, and the other is the exclusion of micro-organisms – bacteria, viruses and moulds. Both are largely properties of the very superficial layer of the skin known as the 'stratum corneum'. This stratum corneum is the final product of the epidermis, which in its turn is dependent on the underlying dermis. It consists of a laminated sheet of minute waxy plates laid one upon the other and held together by a special oily cement. Production of the stratum corneum is the whole 'raison d'être' of the skin. The bottom or 'basal' layer of the epidermis contains cells which are continuously dividing and moving upwards towards the surface (Fig 1.1). They themselves change during this migration to become the waxy plates, and this change is largely the result of rapid production internally of a protein called 'keratin'; this whole process of upward migration and maturation is therefore known as 'keratinisation'. Eventually the surface plates are rubbed or blown away, while being constantly replaced from below. The stratum corneum is remarkably watertight, as well as being flexible, rather like polythene. Its surface is dry and inhospitable to micro-organisms, which generally require a moist environment (Fig 1.2). This film is punctured by small channels which allow through hairs and sweat. An oily liquid, 'sebum', also

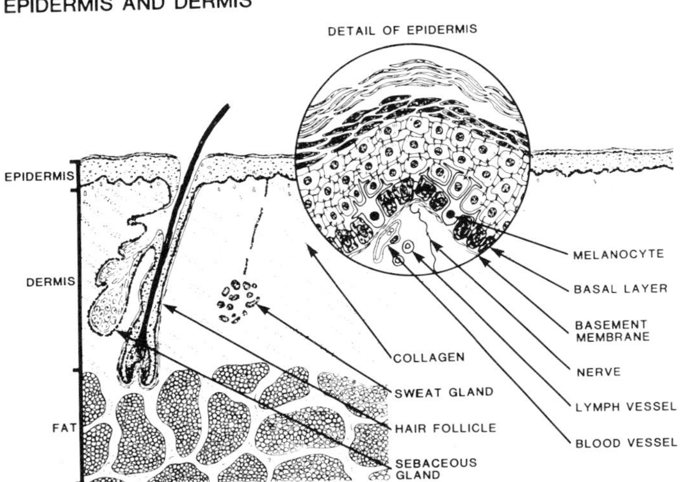

Fig 1.1 Diagram showing the cross-sectional structure of normal skin, magnified.

emerges through the hair channels, and its function appears to be both to lubricate the hair as it slides up through the skin and to add an extra waterproofing layer to the skin surface. The main function of sweat is, of course, to cool the surface by evaporation. On the hands and feet it has a second important job – to help with gripping. As you can imagine, the grip would be very poor if the surface was bone dry.

The underlying dermis is there to support and fix the epidermis, rather as an undercoat does in painting. It consists of a mass of interlacing fibres known as 'collagen', through which run blood and lymph vessels, and nerves. These all end in peg-like 'papillae' which project up into the epidermis. The function of the blood is to supply the oxygen and nourishment needed by the epidermis, and the function of the nerves is to provide the brain with information about conditions on the surface. 'Lymph' is the clear fluid which bathes the tissues. It diffuses out of the blood vessels and is eventually taken up again into a special system of channels known as lymph vessels (see p. 132). These take it back to the bloodstream, but not until it has been passed through special filters known as lymph 'nodes' or 'glands'.

The epidermis is stuck down to the dermis by means of a rather complex membrane known as the 'basement membrane'.

The skin has other functions apart from provision of a barrier. Of these the most important is that of temperature regulation. The skin is analogous to the radiator of a car; it is

Fig. 1.2 The surface of normal skin, magnified 35x, showing the characteristic pattern of ridges and furrows. Droplets of sweat can be seen at the openings of several sweat pores. (Photograph by courtesy of Bencard Allergy Unit, Beecham Research Laboratories).

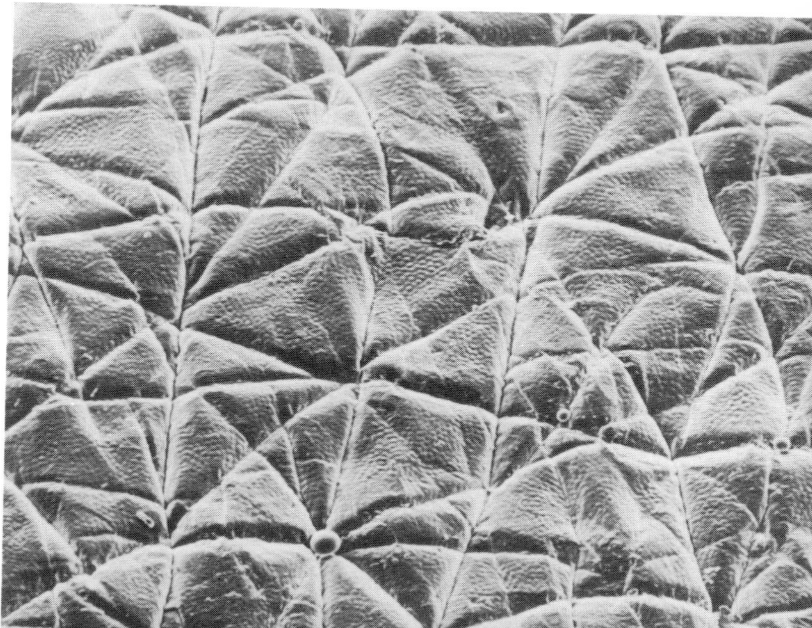

responsible for getting rid of excess heat in order to prevent a rise in the body's heating system. The heating system itself is very much like an ordinary domestic central heating system. The boiler is the liver and the fuel is glucose. The boiler setting may be varied. The pipework is the body's network of blood vessels, and the radiators are the skin. To vary the heat loss the body is able to increase or decrease the supply of blood to the skin. When the supply is great, the skin is red; when it is low, the skin is white, or even blue.

Beneath the dermis is a layer of fat which has two purposes. Firstly, it acts as an insulating layer, to keep the inner core of the body warm when heat is to be conserved. Secondly, it provides a fuel store for emergencies.

So the skin is not just 'hide'; it is just as vital an organ as the heart, lungs or liver. If it is extensively diseased, death may result from serious interference with its functions. Fortunately this is rare, though lesser degrees of interference with function are not all that uncommon. Eczema, when widespread, will, for example, increase water loss through the skin; and parents often remark how much their child seems to drink to make up this loss. Temperature control is another function of the skin which is frequently impaired in children with eczema. They seem to fluctuate wildly between feeling too hot to feeling too cold. The problem stems from excessive heat loss through the inflamed skin. This would lead to a fall in body temperature if there were no compensatory mechanisms. In fact, the body responds in such circumstances by turning up the 'boiler' – that is, by increasing the output of heat by the liver. This requires an increased supply of fuel, which means either eating more or using up stored fat, which can be converted to glucose. This compensatory heat production can, however, cause new problems. If the child now goes into hot surroundings with the boiler turned up, difficulty may be experienced in dissipating this extra heat, because heat loss cannot be greatly increased beyond its already very high level. This difficulty in losing heat is often further aggravated by the fact that sweating is usually impaired in eczematous skin, and the child will now be in danger of overheating. Hence the rapid fluctuations from feeling hot to feeling cold, and vice versa. In old people with widespread eczema these problems can have serious consequences, but fortunately these results of disturbed skin function rarely cause more than discomfort alone in children, though this discomfort may be considerable.

2 What is 'Eczema'?

Eczema is a label which doctors apply to a particular pattern of skin disease. It is just one of many ways in which the skin can react to injury, injury arising either from outside the body or from within. An appropriate analogy would be the car radiator boiling: this is only one of the many problems one can have with a car. Similarly, eczema is only one of many problems one can have with one's skin. A boiling radiator is easily recognised – the problem is to find out *why* it is boiling. There are many reasons why it may have done so, and there are similarly many causes of eczema. Because *people* make cars we understand the way they work, and we can usually pinpoint the problem when something is wrong. Unfortunately, the construction of the human body is much more complex and, since people didn't design it in the first place (thank goodness!), we are at a distinct disadvantage when it comes to understanding exactly how it works and why it sometimes goes wrong. So the analogy ends here.

The kind of eczema we know most about is called 'contact' eczema. It is now recognised that many substances will cause an eczematous reaction if applied to the skin of otherwise normal people, and such substances include acids and powerful detergents. 'Nappy rash' appears to be just such a reaction of young and sensitive skin to urine and faeces. In other cases, contact eczema is caused by an allergy to a normally quite harmless substance such as nickel. This metal is used to make jewellery and fasteners on clothing, and is also used in coinage. Some people become allergic to it and from then on will develop eczema whenever they come in contact with it. The mechanism by which such allergies arise is well established, and we have reliable tests, known as patch tests, to identify them.

Unfortunately we understand much less clearly the causes of other types of eczema. Doctors give different names to the various types of eczema they can recognise, examples being 'seborrhoeic' eczema, 'nummular' eczema and, of course, 'atopic' eczema. To distinguish these varieties of eczema is important because it allows the doctor to know whether he is likely to be able to identify a cause. A good dermatologist will recognise that a gardener with eczema on his face and a patch on one thigh is likely to have developed contact eczema to a chemical in the red tip of a particular brand of matches. The matchbox is kept in the pocket, and the vapour envelops his face when matches are struck. The eczema will be cured simply by changing to a different brand of matches. If a middle-aged man comes to the clinic with eczema consisting of small discs on the outside of the arms and legs, the dermatologist will recognise the pattern as that of so-called 'nummular' eczema (from the Latin word 'nummus': a coin). He knows from this pattern that the man's eczema will not turn out to be caused by any kind of contact and that it will be difficult to cure it permanently with any kind of treatment. The cause of nummular eczema is almost entirely unknown, but it generally tends to disappear after a few years. When a four-year old child comes in with eczema in the crook of the elbows, on the wrists, the backs of the knees and around the ankles, he knows that the child has the type of eczema known to doctors throughout the world as 'atopic' eczema. This disease forms the subject of this book.

3 What is 'Atopic'?

The term 'atopic' is just a name. It actually derives from the Greek word for 'stranger'. Just as the name 'Ford' helps us to identify a particular kind of car, so the word 'atopic' identifies a particular type of eczema. Unfortunately things are a little more complicated than this, because the term 'atopic' is also used to identify a particular type of person. An 'atopic' person is at special risk of developing certain diseases that include 'atopic' eczema, asthma and hayfever; in fact, these diseases are more or less confined to 'atopic' individuals. But how do we recognise such people? By implication, if somebody has one of these diseases that person is likely to be atopic. If they do not, they are going to be more difficult to recognise as atopic, and indeed one would be unable to do so if it were not for helpful tests that have been developed for the purpose. Atopics tend to make excessive quantities of a particular variety of antibody known as immunoglobulin E ('IgE' for short). These antibodies can be detected in several ways, but the simplest in practice is the so-called 'prick test' (Fig 3.1).

In the prick test a drop of a solution containing a commonly encountered substance is placed on the skin. A needle is then pricked carefully into the very outermost part of the skin through the drop, thus introducing a minute quantity into the skin. Antibodies react specifically with the substance against which they have been made. If the skin contains IgE antibody directed against the substance that has been pricked into it, it reacts by producing a weal. The size of this weal can easily be measured and gives some index of the amount of IgE that has been made against a particular substance. The substances used in this test all contain proteins; it is these proteins which react with the antibodies. Proteins which react with antibodies are called 'antigens'. Substances commonly used include house dust mites (small spider-like animals that live in dust), grass

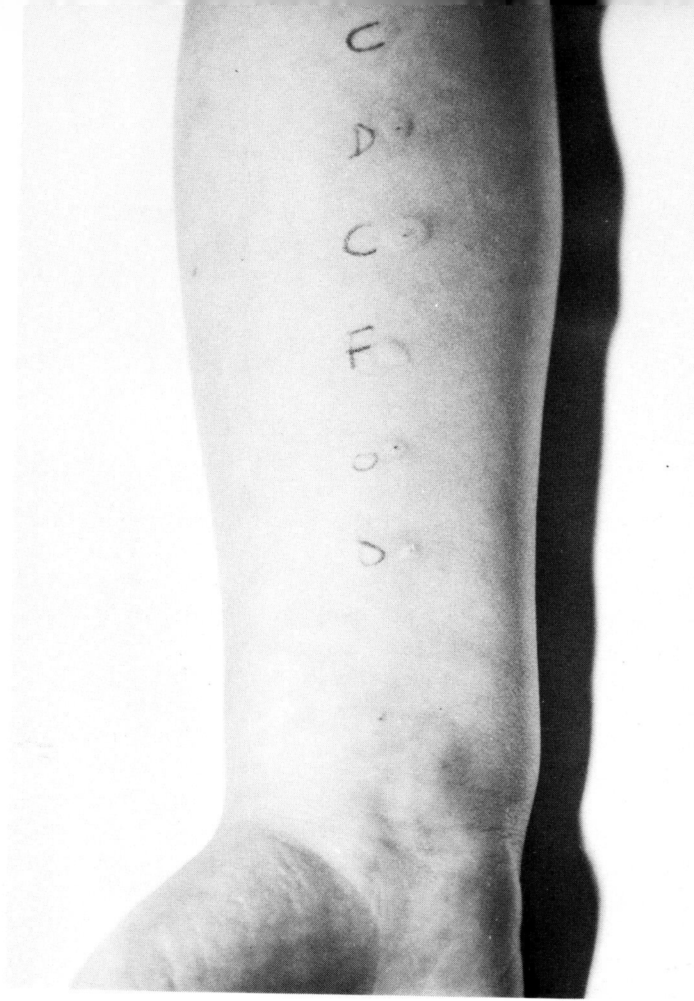

Fig. 3.1 'Prick' tests. These tests are usually done on the inside of the forearm. The point of a fine needle is pricked into the skin through a drop of a substance which is known to be capable of causing allergic reactions. This photograph shows what is typically seen about 15 minutes later, when weals have come up at several of the test sites. The diameter of the weal provides a measure of the degree of allergy present.

and tree pollens, moulds, cat and dog dander, egg and milk. The antigenic proteins in these substances are encountered extremely frequently in our everyday lives.

In practice, as many as a third of all people will produce a positive prick test to one or more substances; all these people are, strictly speaking, atopic. Many will never have eczema, asthma or hayfever, but virtually everyone who does develop one of these diseases will be among this third of the population.

So, atopics are people who are predisposed to develop certain characteristic diseases. They are also people who make abnormally large amounts of IgE antibodies. This does not necessarily mean that they develop these diseases *because* they make these antibodies. Fire engines are red and squirt water; the unwary might wrongly conclude that they squirt water *because* they are painted red, that the magic ingredient is the red paint. We know, of course, that this is not the real reason. The analogy may be relevant to atopics; they get eczema and they make IgE antibodies, but the two are not necessarily cause and effect. Even so, because we know less about eczema than we do about cars, we do not yet understand the relationship between these two facts.

I believe that these concepts are probably the most difficult I will attempt to tackle in this book. If you have managed to follow the discussion so far, the rest will be easy. Before going on, I will try to explain in more detail exactly what 'antibodies' are.

Our bodies need ways to defend themselves against their many natural enemies. Among the worst of these are a vast variety of viruses, bacteria, moulds and parasites, many of which would kill us if given half a chance. We have several types of defence against this bunch of nasties. As well as antibodies, the blood contains special cells called 'lymphocytes', others called 'neutrophils' and yet others known as 'macrophages'; these are known collectively as 'white cells'. The antibodies and white cells are our soldiers, tanks, ships and planes. Just as in the real world, the use of all these different elements of defence requires careful co-ordination. Each element has a special part to play in co-operation with the others, and the loss of any one would result in increased vulnerability. So antibodies are just one of the many forms of defence we have against intruders. They are manufactured by specialised cells known as 'plasma cells' and they react, generally speaking, with proteins, as we have already mentioned. Most of the proteins, of which these viruses, bacteria, fungi and parasites are made, differ from the proteins with which we ourselves are made. The body has ways of identifying these 'foreign' proteins, just as there are ways of identifying other countries' soldiers, tanks, planes and missiles. Once a protein is recognised as foreign – that is, as 'antigenic' – the plasma cells will make antibodies against it. Antibodies are also called 'immunoglobulins' – their chemical name. There are several different types of antibodies, known by code names: 'A', 'E', 'G', 'M' and so on. These different types of antibody have different ways of reacting with foreign proteins. Some form a coating on the protein, making it attractive to the cells known as macrophages, which then eat it up and destroy it – just like sugar-coating a tablet to make it attractive to a child. Immunoglobulin 'E' (IgE) antibodies – the antibodies which atopics make so much of – become attached to yet another group of cells called 'mast' cells. Mast cells contain substances that cause inflammation. Inflammation is rather like an explosion, and mast cells are rather like bombs. The IgE antibody is like a trip-wire attached to a bomb; when disturbed it makes the bomb explode. When a foreign protein meets the right IgE antibody attached to a mast cell it reacts with it and thereby sets off the explosion. The mast cell releases its contents which cause inflammation.

The body has complicated ways of controlling the amounts of antibodies it manufactures. In atopics there seems to be a fault in the control system and, as I have already described, an abnormally large amount of the IgE type of antibody is made.

Antibodies are made against foreign proteins from *all* sources. Foreign proteins are also present in foods, in animals and in plants as well as in viruses, bacteria, moulds and parasites. Although these substances do not actively harm us – unlike the viruses and so on – it is still important to keep them out of our bodies, because the proteins they contain could cause mischief simply by 'getting in the way'.

The atopic state, 'atopy', is inherited; it is passed on from parents to their children. It isn't so much the diseases themselves – atopic eczema, asthma and hayfever – that are inherited, as the predisposition to develop them. This is the reason why parents who have none of these diseases themselves can unexpectedly have a child who does; it is probable that at least one of them is atopic without ever realising it. This is also the reason why parents who had atopic eczema themselves may have children who never get either that condition or asthma or hayfever.

In summary, then, an atopic person is someone who is predisposed to develop certain diseases – the atopic diseases of asthma, eczema, hayfever. If they do not develop these diseases, they may be perfectly healthy all their lives even though they are making unusually large amounts of immunoglobulin 'E' antibodies. Measuring these antibodies is a way of detecting 'atopic' people. Healthy or not, atopics may pass the state of atopy on to their children, who in their own turn may or may not develop these diseases. We will be talking about inheritance and atopic eczema in more detail later.

4 What is Atopic Eczema?

Atopic eczema is largely a disease of children and, in fact, a common one; about 10% of all children develop it at some time. It is a disease of very young children in particular, and three out of four of all who develop this disease do so in the first year of life (Fig 4.1). Curiously, however, it is distinctly unnusual to have atopic eczema during the first six weeks or so, whereas other rashes are common. These other rashes include 'miliaria' (so-called 'sweat rash'), napkin eczema ('nappy rash'), and something known as 'seborrhoeic eczema'. These rashes may be trivial or they may be quite a problem. They are nevertheless all fairly transient and usually get better by the time the infant is three months old. Sometimes the same baby will develop atopic eczema and the one rash may transform

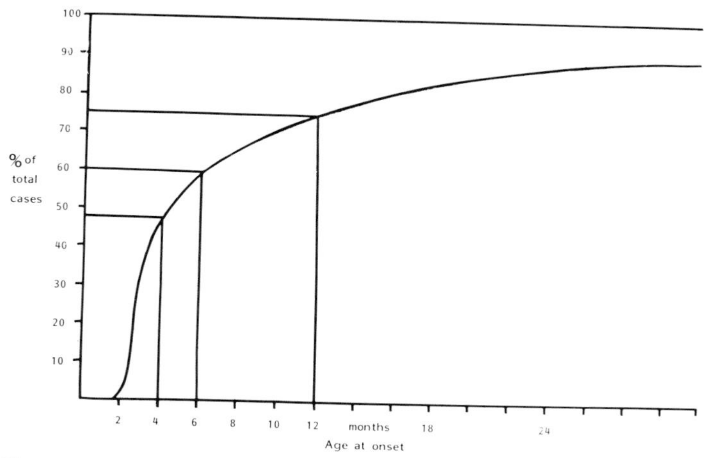

Fig. 4.1. Diagram to show the age pattern of the onset of atopic eczema. You can see that the condition will have appeared by the age of 4 months in some 50% of all those who are destined to develop it, and by the age of 1 year in about 75%.

imperceptibly into the other. It is probably true that babies who have nappy rashes more often develop typical eczema than those who do not. Some of these rashes are rather loosely called 'eczema' by doctors and nurses but the important thing is – what *type* of eczema? Is it *atopic* eczema? The term 'eczema' alone is often used very vaguely.

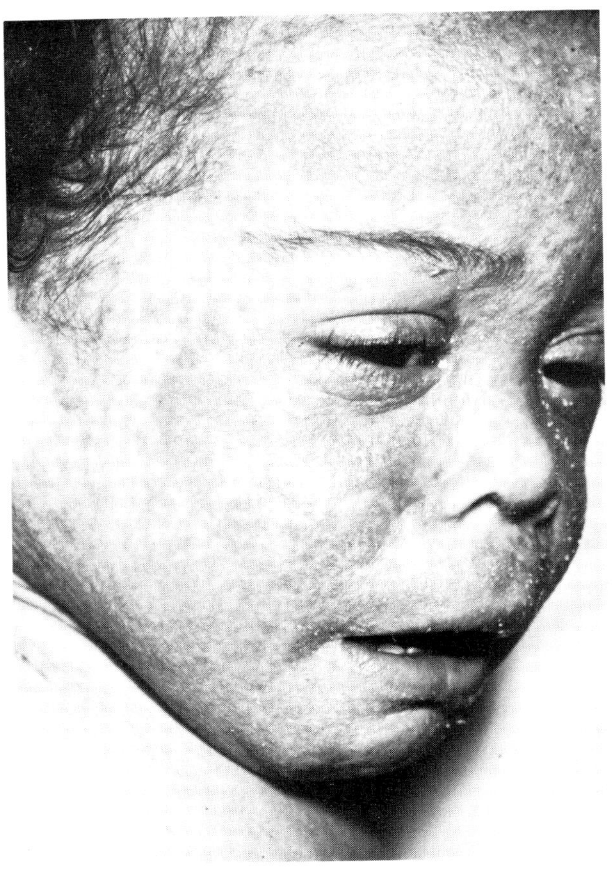

Fig 4.2 Facial eczema. The face is very often the first area to be affected.

Nevertheless, true atopic eczema does not usually develop in this way. Most commonly the baby has good skin until about three or four months old, when an irritating rash starts to appear on the cheeks (Fig 4.2). Quite quickly the rash gets worse, often until the cheeks are raw and weeping. The rash may appear elsewhere, but the face is usually the worst affected

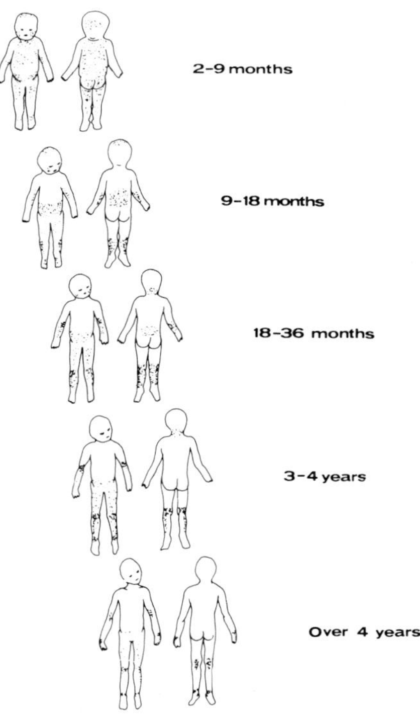

Fig 4.3 Typical patterns of atopic eczema at different ages. Why the distribution of the rash should change during childhood is one of the great mysteries of this condition. Though these drawings show what most commonly happens, in practice the disease can take on an almost infinite variety of patterns.

part of the body at this stage. The constant rubbing of the face on the bedclothes or by the baby's own hands bears witness to the itchiness of the rash. This may now settle down and disappear, or it may gradually turn into more established atopic eczema. If it persists, it tends to progress on to the body and the arms and legs, eventually settling in the creases of the elbows, wrists, buttocks, knees and ankles, (Fig 4.3, 4.4 and 4.5). Why the eruption migrates from the face to the body and hands is a mystery; this is, however, the normal pattern.

Another characteristic feature of atopic eczema is its tendency to fluctuate widely in severity, often for no apparent reason. Later in this book we will consider some of the factors that tend to aggravate or ameliorate atopic eczema, though as often as there seems to be a satisfactory explanation for sudden worsening or improvement of the condition, there seems to be none. Furthermore, the disease affects individual children very differently. In most cases it is fairly mild, no worse than a minor nuisance. In a few, it is severe, disfiguring and disabling. In such cases the disease seems to colour every aspect of the child's life, infecting the parents with despair of an intensity rarely seen in any other childhood disease. In between these two extremes there are children with eczema of intermittent severity.

The hallmark of atopic eczema is extreme irritation; few other skin diseases are quite as itchy. In a child's attempt to stop the itching he (or she) will rip at the living flesh. To the desperation of his parents, nothing will persuade him to abandon his apparent course of self-destruction, and the more effort that is made to dissuade him the more feverishly he tears at the now bleeding skin. At times like this, the child may appear to be in a transported semi-hypnotised state and may seem not to hear or respond to onlookers. This is all extremely upsetting for parents. Undressing always seems to aggravate the irritation and it is often at its worst during the first hour or two after the child has been put to bed. Parents often say to me, 'If only you could do something about the itching, we could live with the rash.' Unfortunately the two are inseparable. If one could

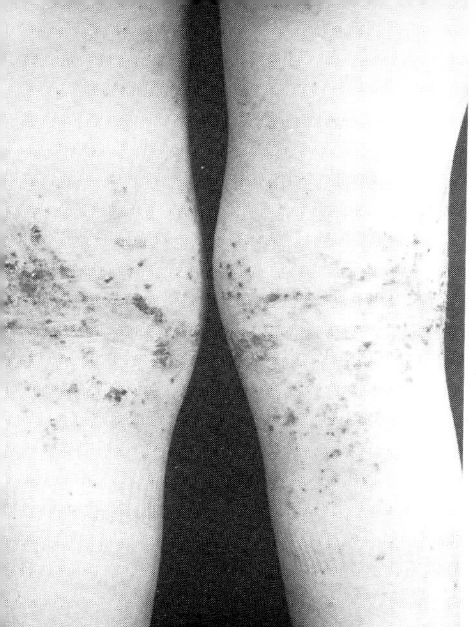

Fig. 4.4 Eczema behind the knees, a favourite site.

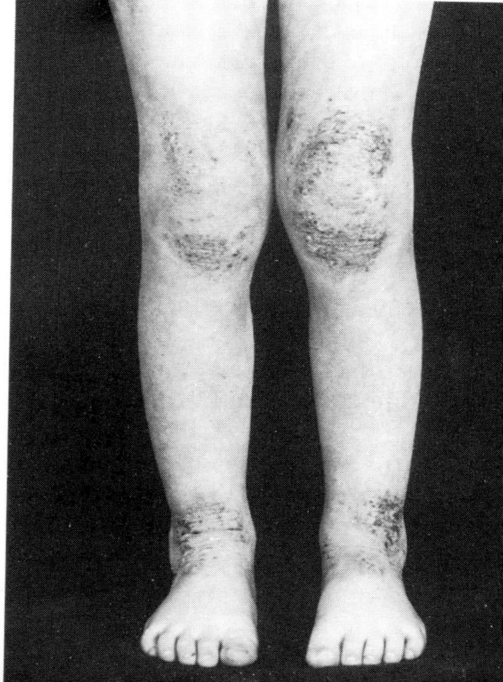

Fig. 4.5 Although the inner aspects of the joints are the most commonly affected areas on the arms and legs, the outer aspects may also be involved in some children. The sites affected in individual children are highly variable.

deal with the itching the rash would be beaten. It has frequently been observed that eczema disappears when a child cannot scratch – for example, when comatose after road accidents, or sometimes when a limb is encased in plaster. Some doctors believe that the disease is really no more than the reflection of a naturally exceptionally itchy skin. All skin has a threshold for itching. Most normal people scratch a little when they get undressed or when they get anxious. Some people are more itchy than others – that is, their itch 'threshold' is lower. Those who believe that atopic eczema simply results from unusual natural itchiness would argue that these children have an inherently low threshold, that they therefore scratch a great deal and that the scratching induces the rash. Personally I cannot believe that this is all there is to it. However much a normal person scratches himself he will not produce eczema, though he will eventually produce 'lichenification', something which we will be considering later. Nevertheless, itching is what can make atopic eczema such a terrible disease, and there can be no doubt that the damage done by scratching plays a major part in producing the damage visible in the skin, even if it isn't the only reason for the rash. In fact, the itching in eczema is probably just another effect of the reaction occurring in the skin which causes the rash. During this reaction, certain chemicals are released within the skin which irritate nerve endings thereby causing the sensation of itch. The interval between the reaction occurring and the worsening of the rash is longer than that between the reaction and the production of the itch. Scratching may therefore precede the worsening of the rash, but this is not because the scratching has caused the rash. Both are results of the same harmful reaction in the skin, a reaction which I will now call the 'eczema reaction'.

The most regular feature of the rash of atopic eczema is redness, for which the medical word is 'erythema' (another Greek word). In some children, the rash never really goes beyond redness plus excoriations – the medical term for scratch marks.

When exacerbations of eczema occur, the first visible sign of this is almost always increased redness. Redness in the skin results from an increase in the flow of blood passing through the dermis (see p. 1). The blood flow depends on the calibre (the internal diameter) of the blood vessels. Increased flow results from an increase in blood vessel calibre ('vasodilatation'). The blood vessel calibre is controlled by chemicals which reach the vessels either in the blood itself or locally from the surrounding tissues. The source of the chemicals responsible for vasodilatation in atopic eczema remains unknown, though it may turn out that they both arrive in the blood *and* are produced locally. I believe that what actually happens is that proteins from the environment first manage to get into the blood and by this route reach the blood vessels in the skin. Having arrived in the skin, they leak out into the surrounding tissue, are then recognised as foreign, and thus initiate the eczema reaction. The chemicals released during this reaction have two effects, firstly they cause itch and, secondly, they increase the calibre of blood vessels causing redness.

The chemicals that cause the skin blood vessels to dilate also make the walls of these blood vessels 'leaky'. As a result of this leakiness, fluid seeps out into the skin from the blood. The result of this is, firstly, swelling (called 'oedema') and, as the fluid penetrates into the epidermis (see p. 1), a bubbly, boiling appearance known as 'vesiculation'. Vesicles are tiny fluid-filled blisters which one can often see looking rather like sago grains just under the skin. This is regarded as the most characteristic of all the features of eczema, and the word 'eczema' actually comes from the Greek word for 'boiling'. When the vesicles reach the surface they are easily broken, either spontaneously or by scratching. The fluid then oozes out on to the surface of the skin, and this is what makes eczema weep (the medical term for weeping is 'exudation'). Because the fluid contains clotting factors from the blood, it can under certain conditions coagulate to form so-called 'crusts', more popularly known as 'scabs' (though this word is now probably best left to its new place in industrial relations language!). The reason why the fluid that oozes out is usually clear rather than bloody is that the red cells in the blood (which give it its colour) are too big themselves to escape from the blood vessels. The increased leakiness of the blood vessel walls makes them like a sieve that lets fluid through but largely keeps particulate matter, like cells, inside. If the blood vessels are more seriously damaged, by scratching for instance, then red blood cells may escape, because there is now a hole in the sieve.

Another feature of eczema is scaliness of the skin. Scaliness is common to many different skin diseases. As we discussed in the introductory chapter, the most important function of the epidermis is to produce the stratum corneum, a waxy protective layer just like the finish on furniture. Normally one is hardly aware of it as it is more or less invisible, although it is constantly being renewed and shed. If at the end of the day you shake out your stockings or socks, the white powder that emerges is the shed waxy material of the stratum corneum. But, just as the finish on furniture can crack and peel if damaged, so can this surface layer of the skin. Scaling occurs when the normal adhesive properties of the stratum corneum are impaired, and this happens in a wide variety of diseases. Children with eczema often seem to have dry scaly skin. Some of this dryness and scaliness is a consequence of the disease. Even in areas where the other features of eczema are not apparent, such as redness and vesiculation, the eczema reaction tends to be occurring to a mild degree deep within the skin. This can be enough to cause the sort of damage that results in scaliness without causing any other visible change. In some families in which eczema occurs, however, dryness of the skin may be common even in family members who do not have eczema. This sort of dryness is called 'ichthyosis' (from the Greek word 'ichthyos', a fish – because in some cases the scaling can resemble the skin of a fish), and this also may be found in families where no-one at all has eczema. It is an inherited condition of the skin which of itself causes little trouble. It seems likely that having this type of dryness of the skin itself also predisposes a person to the development of eczema, but the reasons for this are not clear.

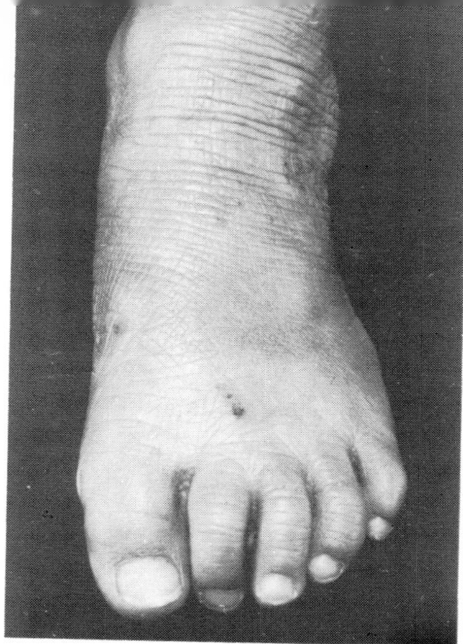

Fig 4.6 In longstanding eczema, the skin tends to become thickened and leathery. This change appears to be a response of the skin to constant rubbing and scratching and is known technically as 'lichenification'.

Eczema is often associated with altered pigmentation in the skin. Skin pigment (melanin) is produced by cells in the epidermis known as 'melanocytes'. People of all colours have the same number of these cells in their skin; the variation in the colour of skin is due to differences in the amounts of melanin pigment produced by these cells. Eczema disturbs the melanocytes, and can temporarily switch off skin pigment production. This effect can be prominent even where the eczema that provokes it is very mild, and in children with a naturally darker skin colour parents may consider it the main problem. Fortunately it is always temporary, though it can last several months at a time in areas of the body from which the eczema itself has disappeared.

The final feature of eczema to consider is a change in the skin known as 'lichenification' (Fig 4.6). The word implies a resemblance to lichen though this may not seem a very apt analogy. If the skin is scratched and rubbed over long periods of time the epidermis gradually thickens. A characteristic feature of this thickening is an exaggeration of the normal skin lines, and the overall appearance may be like leather. This change is common in eczematous areas. Even if the eczema itself clears up, this thickening can last for months and is itchy in its own right. Some otherwise quite normal people have the habit of scratching a particular spot as a sort of nervous release. The scalp, the back of the neck and the shins are common places for this treatment, and eventually patches of lichenification will occur. These itch, and in this way a self-perpetuating cycle of scratching and itching can be set up. Much the same cycle is set up in eczematous children.

5 What Causes Atopic Eczema?

The Allergy Question

The question: 'What is the cause of eczema?' is the one I should most like to be able to answer. As you know, the answer is not known with any degree of certainty, and there are almost as many different views on this as there are dermatologists. My own view is just one of these, but it is shared by some other researchers in the eczema field. I believe that atopic eczema represents a reaction to substances in the environment that are harmless to most people. The reaction appears to represent an excessive and inappropriate response of the immunological system, which is, as we have said, the body's defence system. Excessive and inappropriate reactions of the immunological system to normally harmless substances are known as 'allergic' reactions. People often use the word 'allergy' in a much broader sense to include any adverse reaction to such substances, and especially to foods. This is incorrect; not all harmful reactions to foods are caused by allergy in the strict sense that I have outlined. One must have real evidence that the reaction involves the immunological system. You will remember the sad death of the old king of the elephants in *The Story of Babar* (Fig. 5.1). He was poisoned by chemicals in a mushroom – nothing to do with the immunological system. Here is another example. Parents are usually aware that wool next to the skin will make their child's eczema worse, and at one time it was thought that this might be due to true allergy to wool. But we now think that wool fibres make eczema worse simply by physically irritating the skin; therefore this is not a real allergic reaction.

We have already considered the way the body's defences work in Chapter 2. Its first job is to recognise any foreign protein that succeeds in getting into the body, and its second

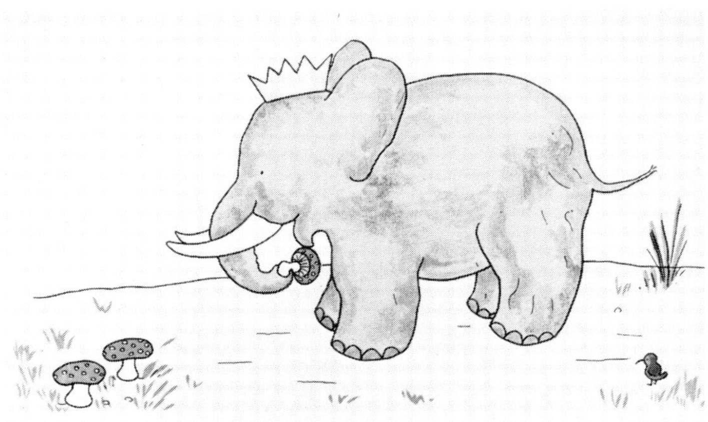

Alas! That very day the King of the elephants had eaten a bad mushroom.

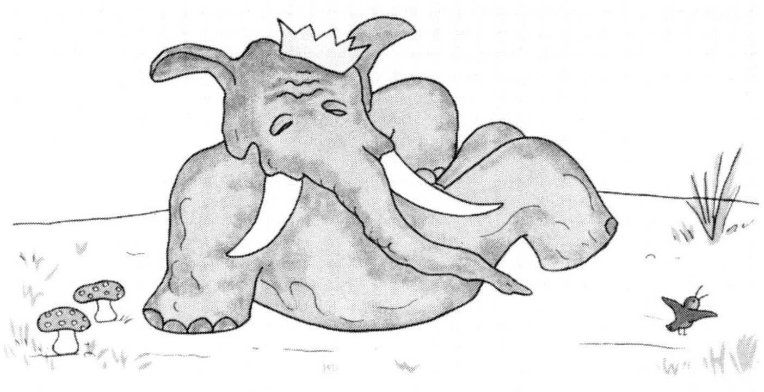

Fig. 5.1 Not all harmful reactions to foods are caused by allergies! From 'The Story of Babar' by Jean de Brunhoff. (Librairie Hachette, Paris, and Methuen, London).

job is to deal with the intruding protein in an appropriate way. Let's use our own country's defence system as an analogy, as we did before. The coastline is under constant surveillance by radar, and by RAF planes and Royal Navy ships on patrol. Any plane that enters our airspace, or any ship that enters our territorial waters, is quickly detected and, if its identity cannot be immediately established, one of our own planes is dispatched to take a closer look. If, on closer inspection, it is decided that the intruder is unwelcome, it will probably be escorted away. But there are other possible courses of action. The intruding plane or ship could be escorted to a home airfield or port, and captured. Alternatively it could be destroyed, or, more aggressively still, the incident might be seen as requiring some more forceful retaliatory action, such as the bombing of a foreign city. Fortunately, in peacetime, the first of these alternative responses is the usual one, and, in this way, intruders are quietly dealt with without provoking incidents. If, tomorrow morning, the RAF responded to an intrusion by an off-course Air India airliner by sending off a squadron of bombers to bomb Delhi, there would be a terrible fuss. The reaction would be regarded by us all as inappropriate and excessively violent. This latter situation is analogous to an allergic reaction, which is similarly excessive in its violence and equally inappropriate to the danger represented by the stimulus.

In my own view, atopic eczema is just such an allergic reaction and I believe that individuals who are liable to this particular kind of reaction are likely to show it as a response to a wide variety of stimuli. You will recall that these stimuli are known as antigens and are foreign proteins. The greatest assault on the body by foreign proteins is provided by the food we eat each day, and it is my own view that foods are of very special relevance to atopic eczema.

Let us consider what normally happens when we eat a meal. The food contains a great mixture of substances. The digestible ones principally consist of proteins, carbohydrates and fats, plus a few extras such as vitamins and metals like iron which we need in very small quantities. The indigestible material largely consists of fibres in plant matter. Digestion takes place in two stages. Firstly the proteins, carbohydrates and fats are broken up into smaller and smaller subunits, rather like reducing a house to a pile of bricks. In the second stage, these smaller subunits are taken up into the blood through the wall of the intestines, a process known as 'absorption'. Since it is proteins that are important from the immunological point of view, let us now focus our attention on what happens to them. Still using the same analogy, imagine you have been given a house which does not suit your needs. It is made of bricks. You want to use the bricks to make a house to your own personal design, totally different from the house you have been given. So you demolish the house you have been given in order to get thousands of separate bricks with which to build the house you want. When you eat the protein in, say, beef, this protein is taken apart and separated into thousands of subunits called 'amino-acids'. These amino-acids pass across the intestinal wall into the blood. From the blood they can be taken up into cells all over the body and used as the building bricks to make a great variety of proteins to your body's own particular design.

The actual amount of intact protein entering the blood after each meal is very small indeed, but is nevertheless enough to stimulate the body's defence system. One way the defence system reacts is by producing antibodies against these food proteins that manage to get in through the intestinal wall. These antibodies link up with the proteins with which they have been designed to react, and thus form what are known as antigen-antibody 'complexes' or 'immune complexes'. These antigen-antibody complexes are gobbled up by special cells which are present in large numbers in certain parts of the body, particularly in the liver, the spleen and the lymph nodes. Such cells are known as 'macrophages'. Once gobbled up by the macrophages, the complexes are dismantled into amino-acids, just as should have happened in the intestines. This sequence of events probably occurs naturally every time we eat anything, quietly and without being at all aware that anything is wrong. It seems that the eczema sufferer's body simply cannot do these things in the same efficient way. The amount of intact food protein entering the blood after meals appears to be greater in those with atopic eczema and the reaction to these food proteins is an altogether more violent one, the end result of which is eczema. The eczema patient makes antibodies against the food proteins, but these antibodies seem to be different from those made by ordinary people. When the antibodies join up with the proteins they again form antigen-antibody complexes, but these complexes are not so attractive to the macrophages and they are not so efficiently removed from the blood. The complexes seem to end up in the skin, where they escape from the blood and then cause irritation and eczema.

It has been suggested that the reason why children get eczema in the first place is because their intestines are excessively permeable to food proteins. The theory is that the normally small amounts that enter the bloodstream in most children lead to development of the safe disposal mechanism, whereas the larger amounts that enter when the intestines are too permeable simply overwhelm the system. The result of this onslaught is that these children cannot develop the normal mechanism for handling such proteins, and instead develop a harmful type of response in the form of eczema. This theory is an attractive one, and there is a certain amount of evidence to support it.

It is unlikely that food proteins are the only ones that could set up this chain of events leading to eczema. Almost certainly many other normally harmless protein-containing substances can do the same thing. Among these the most troublesome include pollens, house dust and animals. The most notorious are the grass pollens (Fig 5.2), presumably because of the vast quantities that are produced. Although we think of pollens mainly as a cause of hayfever they can cause asthma, and almost certainly eczema as well. Although pollen largely reaches the body in the air, very little of the pollen we breathe in actually gets into the lungs. This is because the lining of the air tubes leading down into the depths of the lungs is provided with millions of little hair-like projections that move in a co-

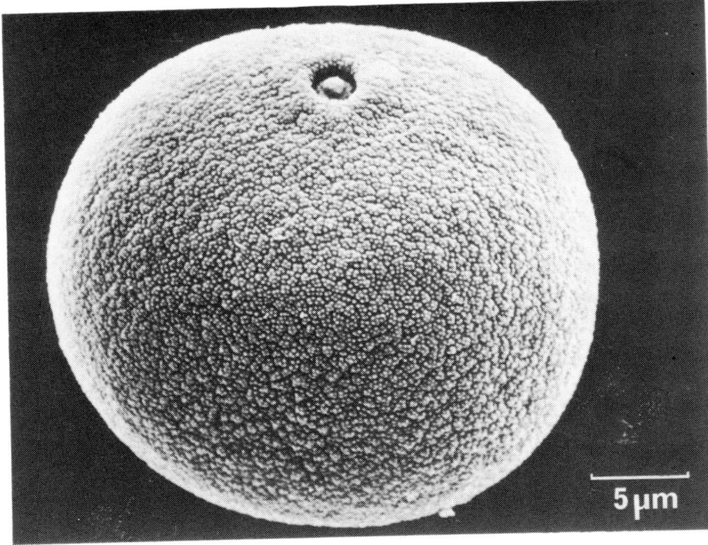

Fig 5.2 A grass pollen grain magnified 4,500x. This is from Timothy grass, the pollen most likely to provoke allergic symptoms in the UK. (Photograph by courtesy of Bencard Allergy Unit, Beecham Research Laboratories).

ordinated way to keep a surface film of liquid moving upwards from the lungs, to the point where the main air-pipe reaches the gullet at the back of the throat. Any particles the size of pollen grains that are inhaled get trapped in this sticky film of liquid, known as mucus, and are then wafted upwards again, finally to end up in the stomach. As a result, in the season, we actually 'eat' a great deal of pollen each day. In the intestines this pollen is dealt with exactly as if it were food. Worse still for the eczema sufferer, the supply of pollen to the intestines is more or less continuous, both day and night, unlike food which arrives only intermittently.

People are often surprised to learn that ordinary house dust contains a very high proportion of human skin scales, which form the staple diet of a tiny creature known as the house dust mite (Fig. 5.3). It is now clear that this animal and its excreta play an important role in causing asthma, and it almost certainly is often responsible for eczema. The house dust mite is particularly comfortable in carpets, sofas and mattresses, and it is ironic that the particularly large amounts of scale produced by eczematous subjects serve as a special encouragement to the house dust mite. It has been shown that the environment of the eczema sufferer is much more densely populated with this creature than that of the normal person.

Pets and other domestic animals are other important sources of antigenic proteins. The shed skin or 'dander' of such animals, or their dried-up saliva, are the main offenders, and

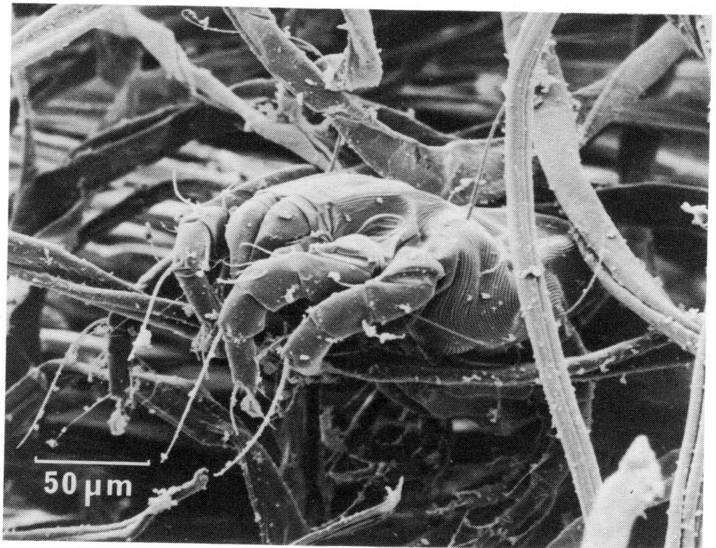

Fig. 5.3 A house dust mite (*Dermatophagoides pteronyssinus*) among fibres of clothing, magnified x450. (Photograph by courtesy of Bencard Allergy Unit, Beecham Research Laboratories).

these substances add to the antigen content of house dust, in addition to the infamous house dust mite.

It seems entirely reasonable, on currently available evidence, to regard atopic eczema as an allergic reaction to any combination of a wide variety of antigens entering the body primarily through the intestine. Nevertheless, there can be little doubt that substances coming into *direct* contact with the skin can aggravate the situation, though there is equally little doubt that atopic eczema cannot be caused by direct contact alone. Substances coming into contact with the skin can aggravate eczema by non-allergic as well as by allergic mechanisms. We will be considering the non-allergic mechanism later on, and for the moment I want to consider the allergic side in isolation, although in practice the two may be difficult to distinguish. A variety of antigens will produce wealing in children with eczema, if introduced directly into the skin in the prick test. This test involves breaking the skin, though the same antigens may produce wealing if simply placed on an unbroken skin on highly sensitive individuals. This seems to be the mechanism underlying the wealing that is seen around the mouth following contact with certain foods in some eczematous children. However, contact reactions to foods are unlikely to be very important aggravators of eczema unless the responsible food is spread around liberally, something which will tend to happen only in very small children. Those antigens which lie around in dust and which land on the skin from the air are almost certainly more important in this respect. Contact between this type of antigen, house dust mite and pollen for example, and eczematous skin, could lead to greatly increased irritation, which in its turn would lead to increased scratching and the introduction of still more antigen into the skin.

In summary, I believe that atopic eczema is the manifestation of an allergic reaction to common substances encountered in our environment, among which foods and airborne substances such as pollen and house dust are particularly important. Proteins from these substances enter the blood both in normal people and in those prone to atopic eczema. In the normal person these proteins are quickly and harmlessly removed by the joint efforts of antibodies and macrophages. In the individual with atopic eczema, the proteins are instead deposited in the skin, where they set up an inflammatory eczematous reaction.

The Role of Infection

Broken, damaged skin provides an attractive environment for many types of micro-organisms, particularly bacteria and yeasts. A few bacteria and yeasts can be found on the skin surface in entirely normal people and, as long as the skin remains healthy, do no harm. They cannot multiply to any extent because the normal skin surface is an inhospitable place. It is dry and covered with inedible waxy scales. But any break in this covering will provide the moisture and nutrients they so badly need, allowing them to proliferate. Multiplying micro-organisms are a potential threat because they compete for the very nutrients that our own cells require; furthermore, under these favourable conditions, they produce a variety of poisonous chemicals known as 'toxins'. There is always the danger that they will actually invade the body, with potentially fatal consequences. The function of the immunological system is to prevent this happening. Wherever such micro-organisms flourish, the immunological system will be at work eliminating them. Eczematous skin provides ideal conditions for many bacteria and yeasts to flourish, and is a terrain in which the immunological system finds it difficult to fight effectively. The result is, at the best of times, a new balance between the micro-organisms and the immune response in which larger numbers of micro-organisms are present while the situation is still kept under some sort of control. In practice, the balance tends to be a rather uncertain one, with the numbers of micro-organisms sometimes being controlled and at other times not. Infection occurs when the number of potentially harmful varieties increases to the point at which the skin is actually damaged by their activities. Infections are among the commonest causes of exacerbations of eczema, and are frequently unrecognised as such. This is a subject to which we will return in Chapter 6, when we consider treatment.

Recently we have started to ask whether these micro-organisms might also play another, more subtle, role in eczema. Bacteria, yeasts and their products contain antigens and it is these which provide the stimulus for the immune response. It is presumably possible for a child with atopic eczema to develop an allergic response to these antigens just as easily as an allergic response is mounted to food and other antigens. The result would be an inappropriate response to these micro-organisms and probably be of the wealing type, which is of course itchy. It would therefore provoke scratching, helping to extend the very environment which is so attractive to the micro-organisms themselves.

The Role of Irritants

The skin of anyone with atopic eczema tends to be unusually sensitive to a variety of irritants. This irritability will be a feature of their skin whether or not eczema is actually present at the time. It is therefore a more or less permanent phenomenon and frequently of lifelong duration. It is somewhat analogous to the irritability of the lungs observed in asthmatic children, in whom asthma attacks may be precipitated by chemicals such as sulphur dioxide (a major industrial air pollutant), paint fumes and even fresh cold air. The term 'irritant' implies a directly harmful effect that has nothing to do with allergy.

Chemicals

A great variety of chemicals seem to be able to provoke or exacerbate atopic eczema after contact with the skin. On the whole they are substances which would irritate the skin of perfectly normal individuals, but the eczema sufferer seems to be especially sensitive to them. Probably the most important chemicals of this kind are soaps and detergents because of their widespread use. The function of both these substances is to remove fats and oils by emulsifying them, and they are very effective at removing these from within the skin. This process is harmful because the oils and fats are there for their protective properties; their removal leaves the skin dry and vulnerable. Soaps are generally milder than detergents, and many manufacturers add fats and oils to their soaps to try to minimize their drying effect. Baby soaps are made with a particularly high content of fats and oils, and are therefore less likely to dry out the skin. So-called 'housewife's hands' are hands dried out by detergents. In some housewives this goes further, and they develop full-blown eczema on their hands as a result of excessive detergent exposure, even if they have never previously had skin problems. But the housewife who has had atopic eczema in the past is especially susceptible. Children with eczema may suffer a great deal from the misguided use of soap on their already inflamed skin. Although baby soaps are less harmful, they should nevertheless be avoided as far as possible.

Contact between inflamed skin and water is initially painful, and for this reason many parents avoid bathing their eczematous children. Paradoxically, water can have a drying effect. Even without the added effect of soap, it can leach out some of the salts and minerals in the skin and can remove some of its oils. Many dermatologists also take the view that bathing is harmful in eczema and advise against it. I take the opposite view, that although bathing with water and soap, or even water alone, may be harmful, the bath is an important component of a comprehensive approach to treatment. Getting water into dry eczematous skin is one of the aims of treatment, but this water must be sealed in by oil. The bath can be used to deliver both this water and oil seal to the skin. I will return to this subject when considering treatment in more detail.

A wide variety of other chemicals can also aggravate or provoke eczema. The following are of special relevance in eczematous children.

Some fruits and vegetables. Many fresh fruits and vegetables are highly acidic, particularly tomatoes and citrus fruits such as oranges, lemons and grapefruits. Contact between the peel or flesh of these fruits and the skin may be highly irritating, and many parents notice that their children get redness and itching around the mouth and on the fingers when eating them. Most of the trouble caused by these foods is probably due to this type of irritant reaction rather than to allergy in the strict sense, though the two can be very difficult to distinguish. Raw onions also tend to be highly irritating to the kin.

Salt. Salt is probably the usual reason for the skin reaction that parents often report around their child's mouth after Marmite or Bovril. Again, it can be difficult to be certain that such reactions are not allergic, but I suspect that direct irritation is much commoner.

Antiseptics. Antiseptics are chemicals that kill bacteria and it is hardly surprising that they tend to be harmful to human cells. Some are highly irritating when they come in contact with the skin, particularly in concentrated form. The widely practised habit of adding antiseptics such as Dettol to the bath is injurious to eczema-prone skin.

Solvents. Solvents are fluids that dissolve other chemicals. Those used in the home tend to be potent lipid-solvent – they swiftly dissolve fats and oils. Skin contact with such solvents leads to the removal of protective fats and oils and this is harmful, just as it is in the case of detergents. Commonly used domestic solvents include dry-cleaning fluids, paint-thinners and strippers, petrol, paraffin and aerosol propellants.

Fibres

The skin is constantly in contact with a wide variety of natural and manmade fibres in clothing, bedding, soft furnishings and carpets. Pure wool tends to be very irritating to the skin of children with eczema and for many years it was thought that they were allergic to it. We are now fairly confident that the irritation is due not to allergy but to some physical property of the fibres themselves. Pure nylon can have a similar harmful effect, and these materials should therefore never be worn next to the skin. Even the small area of contact that may occur where the pullover overlaps at the wrists should be carefully avoided. Pure cotton seems to be the ideal material to wear next to the skin, but it is difficult to obtain and expensive. Cotton mixtures are the next best thing. Nylon bedsheets are best avoided. Carpets of all types tend to be highly irritating and eczematous children should therefore play on carpets as little as possible.

Heat, Cold and Sunlight

Some children's eczema is more or less confined to exposed skin such as the face and hands, and one cannot avoid the feeling that environmental factors could be responsible for this distinctive pattern. Important factors seem to include both extremes and sudden changes of temperature. Radiant heat appears to be particularly irritating, and eczematous children should avoid prolonged exposure to bright sunlight or open fires.

Conditions that induce sweating, including exertion, are frequently a special problem. It appears that sweat cannot flow properly up the sweat ducts in eczematous areas. As a result of damage to these ducts, much of the sweat can leak into the skin instead of flowing to the surface; this leaking of sweat is highly irritating.

Cold winter winds also seem particularly harmful but this is mostly because of their drying effect and is discussed below.

Sudden changes of temperature often initiate itching in eczematous children – on coming into a warm house in cold weather, for example, or undressing.

Low Humidity

Conditions of very low humidity are drying to skin and therefore aggravate eczema. To gain insight into this factor one needs some understanding of the physics of air humidity.

Warm air can carry more moisture than cold air. When cold air cools down, therefore, a point is reached at which the moisture will start to become visible. This is the basis of the formation of dew outside, and condensation inside. The air on a hot summer day in England tends to contain a good deal of moisture, whereas the air on a very cold day in winter contains very little, even if the weather is wet. Below freezing point the air will be exceedingly dry. When this air is heated up inside a house the drying effect is increased because heated air tries to draw up more water than cold air. This means that humidity tends to be at its lowest in well-heated houses in winter, especially when it is dry or freezing outside. Increasing humidity with humidifiers or indoor plants can help, though it also suits house dust mites, and the benefits therefore have to be weighed against the disadvantages. If full anti-mite precautions have been taken, it probably is worth humidifying the child's room in the coldest part of the winter.

The Role of the Psyche

The influence of the mind on atopic eczema cannot be underestimated. Psychological factors play a major role both in maintaining and aggravating the disease, and can probably actually precipitate it in some cases. Conversely, psychological influences can also have a beneficial effect, and this is an aspect to which we will return in a later chapter.

At one time it was thought that children with eczema had a characteristic personality which was itself largely responsible for their developing the disease in the first place. More recently it has been more widely held that any personality trait in an eczematous child is more likely to be a result of the problems caused by having the disease. In fact, there is almost certainly a degree of truth in both of these views.

Observation does suggest that eczematous children are generally more introspective and less extroverted than their non-eczematous counterparts. They seem more sensitive to the emotional stresses of everyday life, stresses which both increase the itchiness of their skin and the aggressiveness of their scratching response. Whereas other children bite their lips or nails, or even pull out their hair as a sign of tension, eczematous children take out their pent-up feelings on their skin. Stresses of whatever cause – being told off, being refused, being bullied, worrying about exams or a place in a football team – are all directed on to the skin. A particular liability to anxiety or to feelings of insecurity does seem to underlie eczema in many children, even in babies, and may well be one of the reasons that such children actually develop eczema. Nevertheless, it is almost certainly true that the rather characteristic personality traits of the eczematous child on the whole arise as a *response* to the disease. Persistent and unpleasant awareness of uncomfortable skin is highly distracting, making it that much more difficult for the child with eczema to take an interest in other people and in other pursuits.

From the emotional point of view, however, an even worse enemy than itching is shame. An eczematous child is not naturally ashamed of his skin, but may be made so by other people. Parents, brothers and sisters, grandparents, schoolteachers and all sorts of other people can do untold emotional harm in this way. Once aware that other people find a child's skin repulsive, any pre-existing tendency to introversion and withdrawal becomes heightened. The stress caused by other people's attitudes, coupled with their own embarrassment, then becomes a potent force in the aggravation of the eczema, and thus yet another circle is established.

In other words, their psychological make-up is simultaneously a result and a cause of their disease.

Summary

The title of this chapter was a simple enough question; 'What causes atopic eczema?' Unfortunately, the answer is not a simple one. In my view, the evidence is convincing that atopic eczema is first and foremost an allergic disease. Children with eczema appear to react abnormally to otherwise harmless substances in the environment, particularly foods and airborne particles such as pollen grains, fungal spores and house dust. This abnormal reaction is expressed as eczema. Because such children tend to react to a variety of these substances, and because there is a delay between exposure and worsening of the eczema, the link between the skin disease and the provoking agents generally remains unrecognised. This is the background, then, upon which other factors are superimposed. Of these, three appear to be of particular importance. These can all aggravate eczema, though they are probably not capable of inducing eczema on their own. The first of the three is infection, which can contribute to the skin damage in eczema without being apparent. Bacteria and yeasts produce toxins that can harm skin directly and it is possible that any damage is done by allergic reactions mounted against these micro-organisms. The second factor is the harmful effect of a variety of irritants. The skin of atopic eczema sufferers seems to be highly irritable, even in areas where the eczema is not apparent. As a result, a variety of irritants can aggravate a child's eczema; these include fibres, chemicals and climatic factors. The third factor is the psyche. In eczematous children, the skin becomes the focus for emotional stress of all types and, unfortunately, the eczema is itself a major cause of such stress.

At any one point in time, a child's eczema reflects the total effect of all these interplaying factors. Allergy appears to be the fundamental cause, other factors being unable to sustain eczema on their own. But, as contributory factors, they can nevertheless exert profound effects on the course of eczema in the individual case.

6 What is the Outlook?

Childhood atopic eczema has a natural tendency to gradual spontaneous resolution after a period. The problem is the great difficulty experienced in trying to predict precisely when this will happen in the individual case. What one can do is to look at the statistics for large groups of children. Unfortunately, what actually emerges is wide disagreement between the findings of different surveys, and this largely reflects the fact that in each survey the researchers were asking different questions in different ways. For example, a group of children known to have had eczema at the age of one can be re-examined, say 10 years later. Some will appear still to have eczema; the eczema in others will appear to have cleared up. Even so, the chances are that some of those who are found to be free of eczema probably do continue to get it from time to time; they just happen to be clear when examined. This will tend to make the outlook seem more favourable than it actually is. Alternatively, one could send out questionnaires asking how the eczema is getting on. Several people will fail to reply, however, and the ones who do so are generally those who still have eczema. This will produce a bias in the other direction and the outlook will seem worse than it actually is.

The typical sequence of events in atopic eczema is as follows: the eczema reaches its worst level over a variable period of time, and then gradually improves until it is clear for most of the time, though it still occasionally reappears. It is actually rather unusual for eczema ever to clear up completely and permanently; most patients go on having some eczema from time to time throughout life, though it may be very little bother to them. The diagram (Fig 6.1) illustrates this typical sequence.

It seems to me that the important question is not, 'When will my child's eczema disappear?', but 'When will my child's

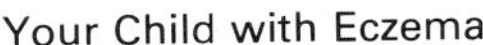

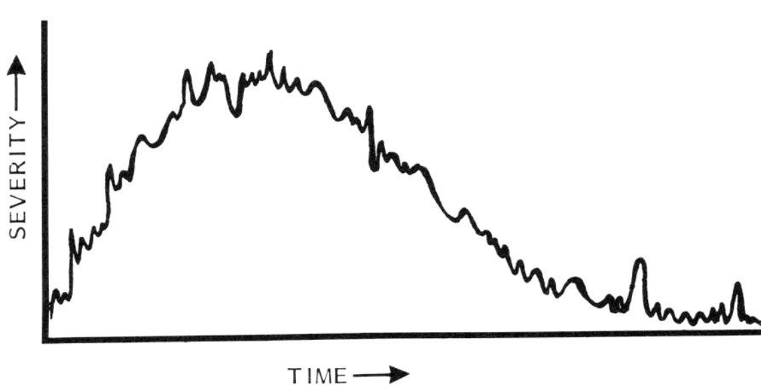

Fig. 6.1 Diagrammatic representation of the typical natural history of atopic eczema.

eczema cease to be a problem?' Despite the conflicting data on this I think one can make some fairly sound generalisations. If a child has eczema at the age of one year there is a better than 50:50 chance that it will have stopped being a problem by the age of five. Of the remaining 50% of children with eczema from the age of one, only about 20% will still have troublesome eczema at the age of 10, and only 5% by the age of 15. Figure 6.2 illustrates the chances of a child who has eczema at one continuing to have problems with eczema at various ages subsequently. As you can see, the curve never quite reaches the bottom of the graph. In other words, there are individuals who will continue to have eczema permanently, and, unfortunately, among these will be a few in whom it continues to be severe. Happily, such individuals constitute only a small minority of those who had eczema in early childhood.

The picture is complicated by the fact that the outlook is also influenced by the age at which the eczema first appears. In general, the later the onset the less favourable the prospects of an early recovery. We have already established that a child with eczema appearing in the first year of life has about a 50% chance of recovery within four years; on the other hand, if the eczema first appears at the age of five, there is probably only a 25%

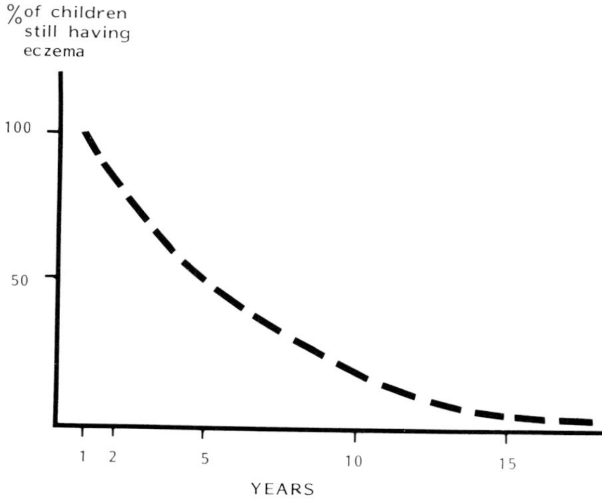

Fig. 6.2 Diagram showing the statistical chances of eczema clearing up in children in whom it initially appeared during the first year of life. You can see that there is about a 50% chance of resolution by the age of 5 years.

chance of the eczema recovering within a further five years, and for a 50% chance of recovery the child may have to wait until the age of 15. I may have been unduly pessimistic with these last figures, but there is no doubt that the outlook is adversely affected by a later onset. If one talks to adults with atopic eczema it is surprising how often the story goes as follows: the eczema was present, but trivial, in early childhood, and subsequently more or less disappeared. But later on, around the age of 10, it reappeared in a more severe form and then persisted.

The course of a person's eczema is peculiar to that individual and therefore completely unpredictable. Any individual may do better or worse than the average. I have given some idea of the overall statistics, such as they are, and they are in many ways fairly comforting. Indeed, a child's treatment must at all times take into account the great likelihood of eventual recovery.

Parents often worry about what their child's skin will be like when the eczema goes. They are usually concerned about possible scarring, and when their child's eczema is severe this is understandable. It is, however, one of the great consolations of eczema that it simply does not scar the skin. This is because the damage occurs quite close to the surface of the skin, however severe it is. This is something that therefore justifies no anxiety whatsoever.

Another type of scarring which parents naturally fear is 'psychological' scarring. They feel that years of eczema cannot fail to take their toll on a child's mental health. Fortunately, this also turns out to be something about which they need not be too concerned. When the eczema clears, most children will quickly forget that they ever had it, even in cases where it has been severe, and they will be psychologically as normal as any other child. Where children do suffer behavioural difficulties later on, these do not generally arise as a direct result of the eczema but indirectly because of the way they have been handled by parents and others. This is why, as far as possible, eczematous children should be treated exactly the same as any other child, why they must never be regarded as 'delicate' or 'different', and why they should *never* be spoiled in compensation for their disease. This is an important subject and we will be returning to it in a later chapter.

I exhort all parents to remember that, however desperate things may seem, in the vast majority of children eczema eventually recovers, and does so without any permanent harm being done either to the skin or to the psyche. This is very different from most of the other chronic diseases that bring children to our hospitals and is something from which to take continued encouragement.

7 How Should Eczema be Treated?

In this chapter I will attempt to consider the range of treatments available for childhood eczema. The difficulty is to find the ideal balance for the individual case. Each eczematous child is different, both in the quality and quantity of the problem, and treatment must be tailored to fit the needs of that individual. Eczema must be neither undertreated nor overtreated. It can be difficult to be sure initially what will suit a particular child, and the ideal treatment combination is often arrived at only by a long process of trial and error. Even then, what is 'ideal' keeps on changing. Only rarely is complete eradication of eczema a realistic therapeutic objective. What one hopes to achieve is a degree of control over the condition. To achieve this control requires a co-operative effort on the part of parents, doctor and child. It is not fair to place full responsibility for treatment on your doctor, and you may lose his support by demanding miracles which he cannot possibly perform. Parents share responsibility for treatment, and its success depends much on their efforts. They must take much of the credit when treatment is successful, and must ask themselves if they do not deserve at least some of the blame when it is not.

I see the function of this small book mainly as one of information. I want parents to share what is known about eczema and how to cope with it. It is worth reflecting that if we really knew all there was to know, there would be no need for this book at all.

The Bath

Parents are often given confusingly conflicting advice about the value of bathing. Some doctors tell them not to bathe their child, or at least to do so not more than once weekly; while others, like myself, tell them to do so every day and, if possible, twice daily. What can one make of all this? It is to some extent understandable why this confusion has arisen. As we have already considered, water and soap alone can be quite harmful to eczematous skin and normal baths should undoubtedly be avoided. The fact remains, however, that the skin of eczematous children tends to be dry and it can be soothed quite markedly by the provision of moisture. What it needs is water which can then be 'locked' into the skin. The best way to do this is by applying a relatively impermeable covering of oil after soaking the skin in water. There are several ways of achieving this, no single one of which is right for every child.

The simplest approach is to add an oil to the bath water. Alpha Keri and Oilatum Emollient are good examples. These are liquid preparations containing either mineral oil and lanolin (Alpha Keri) or mineral oil alone (Oilatum Emollient); in either case 15 – 30 ml should be poured into the bath as it is being run. Another approach is to use emulsifying ointment (unguentum emulsificans). Emulsifying ointment is manufactured by mixing fat with a little detergent; the result is that in water it will 'emulsify' (disperse into small droplets). It does this much more readily in hot than in warm or cold water. It may be emulsified before adding it to the bath water; this is best accomplished by putting two heaped tablespoonfuls in a pyrex bowl, and then adding boiling water straight from the kettle. Whisking will produce a creamy liquid which should be poured into the running bath. This method is ideal for babies in baby baths. In the large volume of a full-size bath this amount of emulsifying ointment tends to make little impression. An altogether simpler way of applying emulsifying ointment is to use it just like soap. Once your child is in the bath, take a good lump into your hand or onto a sponge or flannel, stand your child up and massage it into the skin generally, concentrating particularly on eczematous areas. Rinse it off, and then repeat the cycle two or three times.

When using a baby bath my own preference is to disperse

emulsifying ointment before adding it to the bath. For older children I believe that a combination of an added oil such as Alpha Keri or Oilatum Emollient and emulsifying ointment used as soap is ideal.

A wide variety of other creams and ointments may be used as soap substitutes in exactly the way I have described for emulsifying ointment. The best for this purpose are water-dispersible preparations such as aqueous cream, E45 cream and Unguentum Merck; I particularly favour the last of these for use in the bath.

A few years ago a popular remedy for eczema was to run the bath water through a muslin bag containing either oats or bran. The resulting bath was found soothing to inflamed skin. A range of preparations (Aveeno) have recently become available which revive this approach. They consist of sachets of colloidal oat extract, either with (Aveeno Oilated) or without (Aveeno Colloidal) added oil, and there is also a solid bar (Aveenobar) which looks and works like soap, but contains none. Aveeno-bar is quite an effective cleaning agent and is ideal where something is needed to do the job of soap. It will clearly be impossible to use bath additives if a shower is preferred. Emulsifying ointment can be massaged into the skin during a shower, and the other water-dispersible creams such as Unguentum Merck can also be used. Alternatively, oils such as Alpha Keri and Oilatum Emollient may be applied directly to the skin in the shower.

Lotions, Paints, Creams and Ointments

These are all applications for treatment of the skin, but they differ in their physical properties.

Paints are solutions of aniline dyes such as brilliant green, magenta and crystal violet. These dyes are antiseptic, and solutions containing them can be very useful in 'drying up' weeping areas of eczema. A preservative such as phenol is generally added so that they will keep well over fairly long periods.

Lotions are suspensions of oil droplets in water. Because they provide such an attractive environment for bacteria and yeasts, they must contain preservatives. Even then, once opened, their useful life is very short – maybe only one or two weeks. Like paints, they tend to be rather 'drying' in their effect on the skin. *Creams and ointments* are both quite different from paints and lotions and from one another. Creams are suspensions of fat droplets in water (that is, thick lotions), whereas ointments are either suspensions of water droplets in fat, or just fat alone. Creams, like lotions, are attractive to contaminating micro-organisms, and for this reason do not keep as well as ointments in spite of containing preservatives. These micro-organisms can include ones which cause infections of the skin, and they may initially be introduced into the cream by the person using it. Micro-organisms do not thrive in the fatty environment of ointments, which therefore do not contain preservatives and have a long shelf-life. But ointments are also preferable for other reasons. Being greasier, they work better and also have the advantage of a longer duration of action because they are less easily removed from the skin. They therefore require less frequent application, twice daily generally being more than adequate.

I shall now consider in turn the following types of preparation: moisturisers; corticosteroids; tar; antiseptics and antibiotics; and others.

Moisturisers

Eczematous skin tends to be dry and needs moisture. The drier it is the more moisture it needs. All moisturisers work in the same way. They provide a relatively impermeable surface film of oil which prevents the escape of water from the skin. Because the superficial layers of the skin are damaged in eczema, moisture is lost too rapidly, causing the skin to become dry, stiff and liable to painful cracking. Dried-out skin is also more itchy. Moisturisers ('emollients', in medical language) can reverse the process by replacing the water ('hydration'), and then keeping it in in the same way that the surface layer of the skin would normally do. The film of fat also helps by providing a 'barrier' which protects the skin against the external irritants we have already considered. A wide range of moisturisers is available and most can be purchased across the counter, in addition to being prescribable. They vary greatly, the principal differences being in the proportion of fat to water. This is a list of some of the most popular moisturisers in approximate order of increasing greasiness:

Aqueous cream BP
E45 cream
Oily cream BP
Aquadrate
Ultrabase
Unguentum Merck
White soft paraffin

The more watery moisturisers are often preferred because they leave the skin less sticky, though for this reason they also work less effectively and their benefits tend to be temporary. The greasier ones work much better, but they do tend to leave an obvious oily film on the skin. Nevertheless, they are the ones I prefer. A lot depends on the natural oiliness or dryness of a child's skin. Unguentum Merck has the advantage among the greasier preparations of being water-dispersible – so it can easily be washed off the hands, for example. Aquadrate has a somewhat different way of working: it contains a natural chemical, urea, which rapidly penetrates the skin fairly effectively without being too greasy. Unfortunately, the high concentration of urea can occasionally sting. Calmurid cream is another preparation containing urea, but it tends to be even more likely to 'sting' than Aquadrate and is therefore more useful in other conditions where the skin is dry than it is in eczema. Lacticare lotion is a new product which contains lactic acid. Lactic acid is another natural chemical which attracts water. It also has the frequent side effect of 'stinging' and may turn out to be more useful in other diseases where the skin is dry but less irritable.

Moisturisers are best applied immediately after bathing, when the water content of the skin will be greatest. However, nothing but good can come from frequent additional applications throughout the day, even hourly if possible, especially on exposed areas such as the face, wrists and the backs of the hands. When children are old enough, it is often a good idea to provide a supply of their own to use at school or whenever they like.

Occasionally a child is brought to see me with the story that he or she is 'allergic' to creams and ointments. In actual fact, it is very rare for children to become allergic in the true sense to applications for their eczema. The development of true allergy can be tested for by 'patch tests', in which the material in question is applied to the skin under a dressing and removed after 48 hours. If the child is allergic, a patch of eczema will appear which will still be there a further 48 hours after the test substance has been removed. This sort of test is almost always negative in eczematous children. What actually seems to happen is that the skin in these children has developed an unusual intolerance to grease and oil, perhaps because of blockage of the openings of sweat glands and hair canals. Although this situation does not reflect genuine allergy, it can nevertheless cause real problems when treating the affected child.

For similar reasons a particular product will not always suit every child and, as I mentioned earlier, this will depend to a great extent on the natural texture and oiliness of the child's skin. It is very difficult, if not impossible, for the doctor to choose the ideal preparation first time every time, and finding it tends to be a process of trial and error. What is perfect for one child may not suit another at all.

Having said this, there is no question that true allergy to one or more ingredients of creams and ointments does occasionally occur, and the older child or adolescent is at most risk of this complication. The sensitivity is most commonly either to a preservative or to lanolin. The most frequently involved preservatives are ethylenediamine and parabens. Lanolin is a fat obtained from sheep's wool. Manufacturers are constantly seeking to replace these potentially troublesome ingredients and some preparations, such as Unguentum Merck, emulsifying ointment and white soft paraffin contain none at all.

Corticosteroids

In the last few years, a great deal has been written about the dangers of corticosteroids in the treatment of all sorts of diseases; the result is widespread confusion, even among doctors. When they first became available in creams and ointments, it was expected that their use would revolutionise the treatment of a variety of skin diseases, particularly eczema. After the initial unqualified enthusiasm had settled down, it was clear that their use could cause problems if appropriate precautions were not observed. They do, nevertheless, have an important place in the treatment of childhood eczema and, if caution is observed, they may be used with complete safety.

'Steroids' are a group of natural hormones produced in many parts of the body. Those produced by the so-called 'cortex', a part of the adrenal glands (which lie just above the kidneys), are termed 'corticosteroids' because of the site of their manufacture. From there they are secreted into the blood, and thence circulated to the body as a whole. The cortex produces some hormones that influence the reproductive system, and others that influence the balance of salt and water in the body. The principal effect of the corticosteroids which concerns us is a damping-down effect on inflammation, though exactly how this effect is achieved is still not fully understood. When the body is injured, for example by an accident, operation or infection, the cortex responds by increasing its secretion of this type of hormone. As well as having beneficial effects on the injured tissues, these hormones have important effects on bodily function as a whole under conditions of stress by maintaining both the blood pressure and the supply of glucose and nutrients.

When corticosteroid hormones were first given by mouth or

injection for the treatment of disease, it became clear that they could have potentially serious side effects. If they are given regularly, especially for periods exceeding a month, the cortex reacts by closing down its own production of corticosteroids. This is no problem from day to day because only small amounts are needed in normal circumstances, and adequate supplies of hormone are in any case being provided from outside. But the cortex progressively loses its ability to increase its production in response to stress. Normally this increase is many fold. This means that suddenly there may be a deficiency in supply of the hormones; the blood pressure falls and the supply of nutrients to the tissues fails. The result can be sudden collapse, potentially fatal unless the reason is quickly recognised. If anyone has been on corticosteroids by mouth for more than a month they need an increased dose in conditions of stress. Because they may have an accident, and therefore be unable to tell anyone that they are taking this form of treatment, they should carry a card giving this information or, better still, wear a Medic-Alert bracelet or pendant at all times. (Further information available from Medic-Alert Foundation, 11/13, Clifton Terrace, London N4 3JP. Tel: 01–263 8597.) This problem does not occur with corticosteroids applied only to the skin, except in cases of extreme overuse.

The other type of side effect, which is not life-threatening but is nevertheless highly undesirable, results directly from the actions of larger-than-normal amounts of these hormones on various parts of the body. The most important of these is a suppressive effect on growth. After a period, high doses of corticosteroids given by mouth or injection will invariably produce some degree of stunting, due to a dampening effect on the growing parts of the limb bones. Some diseases themselves cause stunting, however, and the stimulatory effect on growth produced by successful treatment may more than compensate for the stunting effect of the corticosteroids themselves. The overall effect can therefore be an actual acceleration of growth. Nevertheless, the net effect of oral corticosteroid treatment will generally be a degree of slowing of growth, though this can be minimised to some extent: (i) by giving the lowest possible dose; (ii) by giving the corticosteroid as infrequently as possible, where feasible only one dose every two days; (iii) by using this form of treatment for the shortest possible period. Small degrees of stunting will often be compensated for by 'catching up' when the treatment is stopped.

These are the main problems associated with the use of oral corticosteroids. In many diseases they provide enormous benefits which cannot be obtained with any other form of treatment, benefits which far outweigh any possible problems. The immense good that can be done by careful corticosteroid treatment is sometimes ignored by their often ill-informed critics in Sunday newspapers and elsewhere. In childhood atopic eczema, however, their use is only very rarely justified, because the disadvantages will generally outweigh the benefits. Unfortunately, relatively high doses are required to control more severe degrees of eczema, and continuous treatment over months or years will usually be needed to maintain control. This tends to mean that side effects will be virtually inevitable. Occasionally their use is justified, but the decision is a difficult one and one that should be taken in conjunction with parents.

An alternative way of giving corticosteroid treatment is to stimulate the child's own adrenal glands to increase their production of these hormones. This can be done by giving injections of 'ACTH', which stands for 'Adrenal Cortex Trophic (that is, stimulatory) Hormone'. Under natural conditions this hormone is produced by the pituitary gland (situated at the base of the brain), in response either to stress or to low blood levels of corticosteroid hormones. It is then carried in the blood from the pituitary gland to the adrenal cortex, where its effect is to stimulate increase production of corticosteroids. The advantage of giving ACTH (usually in the form of a brand called Synacthen) is that it will not suppress the function of the adrenal cortex. There are, however, two disadvantages. Firstly, the response of each individual's adrenal glands to a particular dose is highly variable, so that it can be difficult to know how much effect one is going to get from any particular dose. Secondly, potentially dangerous allergic reactions can occur against this synthetic hormone and, although these are rare, the risk needs to be taken into account. For these reasons, most doctors prefer corticosteroids to ACTH.

Corticosteroids may also be used to treat skin diseases by applying them directly (in medical language 'topically') to affected areas. They are effective when used in this way because of their ability to penetrate to the deeper layers of the skin where the eczema reaction actually occurs. Unfortunately, it is precisely this ability to pass through the skin which may cause problems. A proportion of the hormone applied to the skin will inevitably end up in the blood and, if the amount is great enough, the result will be problems identical to those encountered when corticosteroids are given by mouth. The danger of this happening depends on four factors: (1) the potency of the preparation used; (2) the surface area treated; (3) the amount applied (clearly this is at least partly related to (2)); and (4) the age of the child. Age is important because the smaller a child the greater is the proportion of surface area to weight. In other words, the hormone absorbed from treatment of one square centimetre of a baby will have a relatively greater effect on the whole child than it would on a bigger child. Added to this is the fact that a baby's skin is unusually permeable. A greater proportion of any chemical applied to a baby's skin will end up in the blood than it would in an older child.

Let us now consider in more detail the question of the potency of different preparations. This will depend both on the innate potency of the particular hormone used and on its concentration. The following is a list of commonly used corticosteroid preparations which I have divided into four groups on the basis of overall potency:

1. *Low potency:*	hydrocortisone ½%, 1% or 2½%	(Efcortelan) (Alphaderm)
2. *Low–medium potency:*	clobetasone butyrate 0.05%	(Eumovate)
	fluocinolone acetonide 0.0025%	(Synalar 1 in 10 dilution)
	flurandrenolone 0.0125%	(Haelan)

3. *Medium potency:*	hydrocortisone 17–butyrate 0.1%	(Locoid)
	fluocinolone acetonide 0.00625%	(Synalar 1 in 4 dilution
	fluocinolone acetonide 0.01%	(Synandone)
	betamethasone valerate 0.025%	(Betnovate RD)
4. *High potency:*	betamethasone valerate 0.1%	(Betnovate)
	beclomethasone diproprionate 0.025%	(Propaderm)
	fluocinolone acetonide 0.025%	(Synalar)
	fluocinonide 0.05%	(Metosyn)
5. *Very high potency:*	clobetasol proprionate 0.05%	(Dermovate)
	fluocinolone acetonide 0.2%	(Synalar forte)

In most cases these are available either as cream or ointment and, for reasons which we considered earlier, the ointment form is generally preferable. A reduction in potency of a corticosteroid preparation is commonly achieved by diluting the product in a cream or ointment base, so that the final strength is a half, a quarter or even a tenth of the original. A one-in-ten dilution of Synalar, for example, is approximately equivalent to Eumovate. At one time such dilutions had to be obtained from the pharmacists's slab in the hospital or in the chemist's shop. For various reasons diluted preparations made in this way are unsatisfactory. The strength of the diluted corticosteroid is likely to fall off very quickly, resulting in a lack of effect. Contaminating micro-organisms are likely to be introduced during the diluting process. In the case of corticosteroid preparations containing antimicrobials, the concentration of the antimicrobial agent will usually be reduced below that at which it is at all effective. Several manufacturers now make these dilutions themselves under carefully controlled conditions which overcome these problems, and 'home-made' dilutions need no longer be prescribed. This represents a considerable advance.

There is a definite risk of internal side effects when Group 4 or 5 preparations are used on eczematous children. The risk is greatest when large amounts are used on extensive areas of skin, and is greater in younger children. It is impossible to give reliable guidelines as to precisely what is or is not safe. In practice, most dermatologists now believe that Group 4 or 5 preparations should never be used undiluted for eczema in children of any age for periods exceeding a week. As I have already mentioned, it takes at least two weeks for any danger to appear. It must be admitted, however, that the risk will be minimal if only very limited areas are sparingly treated with such preparations in older children. Group 2 or 3 preparations are unlikely to cause internal side effects except in babies, although Group 3 preparations may do so if used on extensive areas in large quantities over a long period. Group 1 preparations – that is those containing hydrocortisone alone – effectively *never* cause internal problems, unless used extremely injudiciously in very small babies.

Apart from the potential hazards consequent upon absorption of topically applied corticosteroids into the bloodstream, there are two other problems which may be encountered when such preparations are used. The first is their ability to damage the skin; the second is a phenomenon known as 'tachyphylaxis'.

The damage caused to skin by corticosteroids is known as 'atrophy'. This type of damage may be caused by corticosteroids given by mouth, but tends to be more of a problem with topical preparations because the concentration reached locally in the skin is generally higher. Atrophy is similar to what happens to the skin quite naturally as a result of the aging process. It becomes thin, transparent and fragile. These changes are due to thinning of both the epidermis and the dermis, though the effect on the latter is the more profound. As mentioned in the introductory chapter, the bulk of the dermis is provided by a mass of intertwining fibres made of a protein called collagen. In the normal skin, production of new collagen fibres goes on alongside dissolution of old or damaged fibres. Both in old age and under the effect of corticosteroids, the balance of production and dissolution is altered so that new production is inadequate to replace losses and the dermis gradually wastes away. The epidermis loses its support and becomes more fragile. The blood vessels that run in and through the dermis become more easily visible from the surface. During its early phase, this atrophic change is reversible; if corticosteroid treatment is stopped, the skin will return more or less completely to normal. The dermis can, however, become so attenuated that it loses its elasticity altogether; at this stage unpleasant 'striae distensae' ('stretch marks') will appear, just like those often appearing on the abdomen in pregnancy. If this happens, the skin may never again return to normal; striae are permanent.

The rapidity with which atrophy develops depends on the potency of the preparation and the frequency with which it is applied. It also depends on the site to which it is applied. The face is especially at risk and for this reason preparations other than those in Group 1 should, generally speaking, not be applied to the face. The danger of atrophy is a very real one when preparations from Groups 4 and 5 are used though, as always, much depends on how much and how often they are used. Atrophy takes several weeks to develop, and will therefore be avoided if potent preparations are used for no longer than a week at a time. It is therefore perfectly justifiable to employ these preparations for a few days as an emergency measure to cope with sudden flare-ups. If one goes on applying them, however, not only do internal side effects and skin atrophy appear but their effectiveness will also wane as 'tachyphylaxis' develops (see p. 56). This may mean that one is subsequently left with no choice but to use stronger preparations until one runs out of new preparations altogether. For all these reasons Groups 4 and 5 preparations should only in exceptional circumstances be used for longer than one week at a time, with at least a four-week interval between such courses.

Group 2 and 3 preparations will not cause visible atrophy except on the face. Hydrocortisone alone (that is, Group 1 preparations) never causes atrophy, even on the face. It must be apparent by now that hydrocortisone is unique in its margin of safety and, although there is a place for more potent corticosteroids in older children, nothing stronger than hydrocortisone should *ever* be used in babies.

'Tachyphylaxis' is the medical term for a phenomenon that occurs with externally applied corticosteroids, but curiously enough, apparently not with corticosteroids given by mouth. After a period of regular use, any particular preparation will gradually start to lose its effect. How rapidly this occurs depends largely on how often the preparation is used. It will happen more if it is applied twice daily than once daily, and more if it is applied once daily than if it is used only occasionally. When a particular preparation is applied once or twice every day this loss of effect will usually appear after only a few days and will become more and more noticeable after that. It also seems to happen more rapidly with more potent preparations – that is, those in Groups 4 and 5. It can be partially overcome by using it less frequently or, where this is not feasible, by changing to another preparation. Often the best tactic is to change brands within the same potency group every few weeks. After a particular preparation is stopped for a few weeks it will usually be found that it has regained much of its former potency; in other words, 'tachyphylaxis' is reversible. Unfortunately, with the more potent Groups 4 and 5 preparations, it is found that the effectiveness of the whole group wanes with continuous use, even if preparations are changed regularly.

In some forms of eczema in adults, especially in eczema of the hand, the effect of corticosteroid application can be amplified by the use of polythene film. This technique is known as 'occlusion', and it works by increasing the hydration of the skin. Hydration enhances the transport of corticosteroids through the barrier of the stratum corneum, and occlusion will therefore greatly accelerate the rate at which atrophy occurs, when potent corticosteroid preparations are used. This technique is in fact rarely used in children because of the extensive areas which normally require treatment in the severely affected case. A lesser degree of hydration is, of course, achieved by bathing and by using moisturisers, both of which also enhance the permeability of the stratum corneum to corticosteroids applied subsequently. This is an effect on which we depend to penetrate this barrier, and to get any effect at all from the treatment. In fact, all corticosteroid preparations are made up in what is effectively a moisturiser. As we have already said, ointment bases are better hydrators than creams and lotions and therefore work better. This is also the reason why corticosteroids are best applied after the bath. I personally believe it may be best to apply a thin layer of corticosteroid ointment under a more generous application of an emollient such as Unguentum Merck, or white soft paraffin. This helps to provide plenty of moisturising effect without requiring an excessive application of corticosteroid.

Tar

It has been recognised for many years that tar has a soothing effect on inflamed skin, and it is a traditional remedy for several skin diseases including eczema. Tar is a natural mixture of hundreds of chemicals, many of which have medicinal effects. Tars for treatment of skin disease are obtained by distillation from three main sources; coal, bitumen and wood. Coal tar is the type most commonly used in the United Kingdom. At one time it was wide practice to apply crude coal tar direct to the skin. Unfortunately, this crude coal tar could itself be irritating; it is also messy and, cosmetically speaking, a disaster. It is therefore more usual these days to apply it in diluted form as a constituent of one of a wide variety of preparations. It is often made up in an ointment or a paste, and recently some very mild preparations combining tar with hydrocortisone have come on to the market. A popular example of such a mixture is Tarcortin cream. Coal tar is also occasionally added by hospital pharmacies to more potent corticosteroid preparations, and such mixtures are often popular with patients. What is not widely appreciated is the fact that the strongly alkaline tar partially inactivates the corticosteroid and the result may be simply rather an expensive coal tar ointment.

Probably the best way of applying tar to the skin is in the form of tar paste bandages, and these will be discussed in a later section of this chapter.

Bitumen is traditionally obtained from shale deposits containing fossil fishes, and that is why bituminous tars are known by such names as 'ichthyol' and 'ichthammol' ('ichthyos': a fish, in Greek); these tars are milder than coal tars. Wood tars are widely used in Scandinavia but rarely, if ever, in Britain.

Others

A variety of other agents are sometimes used on the skin for treatment of eczema. These include crotamiton, calamine, so-called non-steroidal anti-inflammatory agents, antihistamines and local anaesthetics.

Crotamiton is an agent which has mild anti-itch properties and is available as a lotion or ointment (Eurax), or combined with hydrocortisone in a cream (Eurax HC). These preparations are widely and successfully used in scabies, but in my view have little, if any, role in the treatment of eczema. The occasional patient does seem to like them and they are free of problems, though they may irritate when eczema is in an exudative phase.

Calamine is another substance occasionally used in eczema. Calamine is zinc carbonate, coloured pink by a trace of iron oxide. Calamine lotion is a traditional soothing application which has found its main use in burns, sunburn, insect stings and so on. It has a pronounced drying effect and is therefore inappropriate for eczema in dry phases. It may be used for exudative eczema, but the powder content tends to cause a build-up of lumpy crusts, and it is in any case less effective in these circumstances than the antimicrobial paints and lotions which will be discussed in a later section of this chapter. Calamine is an ingredient of some of the paste bandages we will also be discussing later on.

A large choice of drugs has been developed as an alternative to corticosteroid tablets for treatment of arthritis, and they are therefore known as the 'non-steroidal' anti-inflammatory drugs. Well-known examples of these include indomethacin (Indocid) and phenylbutazone (Butazolidin). These are taken by mouth or administered by suppository. Similar drugs have now been incorporated into preparations for applying to the skin, and the best known of these is bufexamac (Parfenac). These will probably turn out to be safe for use on the skin, but – for the present – the evidence suggests that they are far less effective in eczema than corticosteroids. This is nevertheless a promising line of development, and more effective preparations containing such drugs may eventually become available.

We will be discussing the undoubted value of orally administered antihistamines in eczema in a later part of this chapter. These drugs are also put into various lotions and creams for direct application to the skin, and there is no doubt that they can be fairly good at relieving the sensation of itching in some skin disorders. In eczema they are unfortunately even less effective than the mildest corticosteroids, but their real downfall is a distinct tendency to provoke allergic reactions after they have been used for any length of time. If this occurs in a child with eczema, it can be difficult to appreciate what has happened because the allergic reaction is also eczematous. Worse still, the child will have become allergic to antihistamines and closely related drugs given by mouth as well. This kind of allergy is virtually permanent once it has arisen, and its presence can be quite a serious problem because drugs of this type are used to treat not only eczema but also asthma, hay-fever, rhinitis, urticaria and a wide variety of psychiatric disorders, including anxiety states. Topical antihistamines may be useful in relieving the discomfort of sunburn and insect bites and little risk is attached to their use for these purposes, as these conditions are by their very nature shortlived. Examples of such preparations include Caladryl cream and lotion which contain both an antihistamine and calamine, Phenergan cream and Anthisan. All of these can be purchased over the counter at chemists, and parents may be tempted to buy them. As far as eczema is concerned, however, they are best avoided.

Exactly the same problems arise with local anaesthetics. They do temporarily relieve the sensation of itching, but to maintain this effect requires virtually continuous application, which is associated in the long term with a real risk of allergic sensitisation. As with topical antihistamines it is perhaps unfortunate that so many of these preparations can be bought over the counter. Available preparations include Dermogesic ointment, Locan cream, Nestosyl and Nupercainal. In the case of some topical antihistamines and local anaesthetics, it is stated in the accompanying leaflet that their use is contraindicated in eczema, but these are by no means always provided.

Antibacterials

Antibacterials are substances given either internally or externally to kill bacteria. This group of substances includes both antibiotics and antiseptics. Strictly speaking, antibiotics are chemicals secreted either by moulds or by bacteria themselves to provide protection against other bacteria, but in practice these days the term is used in a broader sense to include all drugs given internally to treat bacterial infections, whether produced by other micro-organisms or wholly synthetic, as many now are. Antiseptics are toxic chemicals that are not only lethal to bacteria but also harmful enough to humans to preclude their internal use.

In Chapter 4, I described how eczematous skin inevitably supports an unusually high population of bacteria and moulds, many of which are capable of aggravating the skin condition if their population reaches a sufficient density. In this latter case, the term 'infection' is appropriate, because it implies that the micro-organisms are definitely having a detrimental effect. The term 'colonisation' is correct for the more common situation where there is a population of micro-organisms, even including potentially harmful varieties, but where there is no reason to believe that they are actually having a harmful effect. *Staphylococcus aureus* (Fig 7.1) is a particular type of bacterium

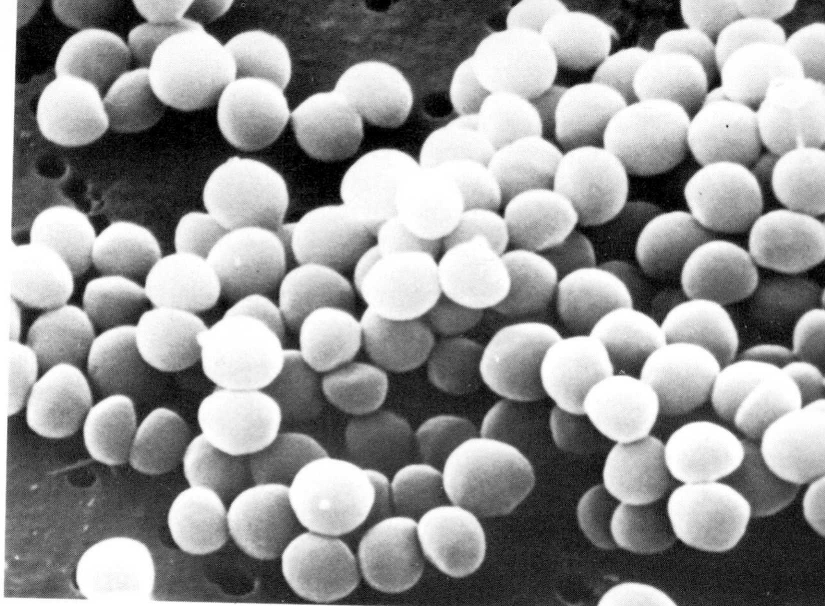

Fig. 7.1 *Staphylococcus aureus* bacteria, magnified x12,000. These bacteria are the most common cause of skin infections in children with atopic eczema. Normal skin is a hostile, uniniviting environment for such micro-organisms, whereas eczematous skin is a very attractive one. (Electronmicrograph by courtesy of the Bencard Allergy Unit. Beecham Research Laboratories).

which appears to be responsible for the great majority of significant bacterial infections in children with eczema. It now seems clear that a population density of over one million of these bacteria per square centimetre is harmful to eczematous skin; that is to say, this population density represents a true infection, whereas a smaller population should be regarded as colonisation only. But how does one detect the presence of infection?

Infection with *Staphylococcus aureus* should be suspected wherever there is exacerbation of eczema associated with weeping and the appearance of either crusts with a particular yellow hue (aureus: golden, in Latin), or pus-filled spots. These changes in the skin are often combined with painful enlargement of lymph nodes and, occasionally, with fever. In practice, it is not always possible to be sure whether a particular exacerbation is caused by infection or not, and it is largely a question of maintaining a high level of suspicion. This bacterium is the same one that causes the highly contagious infection known as impetigo, which occurs in otherwise normal children, and recent contact with such a child would make one especially suspicious. Impetigo often occurs simultaneously in the brothers and sisters, or even parents, of infected eczematous children. When eczematous children are carrying these bacteria, parents may notice that they are getting various skin problems, such as crops of pus-filled spots, boils, or infections in cuts, abrasions and so on.

Unfortunately, infections of eczematous skin by *Staphylococcus aureus* are not visually obvious until their population density reaches ten million per square centimetre, that is, 10 times the population known to aggravate the eczema. This means that harmful infections may not be detectable at all by eye, and special tests would be needed to be certain that this type of infection is present. As you know, doctors often take 'swabs' from the skin if an infection appears to be present. This generally means rubbing a moistened cottonwool ball into the affected area, then sending it to a hospital laboratory. In the laboratory, this material is in its turn rubbed on to a special plate of nutrient jelly known as 'culture medium', and the plate is placed overnight in a warm 'incubator'. The next morning the bacteria will have formed little spots on the jelly, known as 'colonies', just like mould growing on food. The type of bacterium may be recognised by the shape, texture and colour of these colonies, and by looking at the bacteria within them under a microscope. One can get some idea of the population density of the bacteria on the patient's skin from the number of colonies on the culture plate. Nevertheless, the number of colonies appearing will depend on many other factors and this poses a problem of interpretation for the doctor. Bacteria never normally occur in some situations, for example in the blood, and their culture from blood therefore demands action, whatever the number. But in the skin the situation is entirely different. As we have already seen, even perfectly normal skin provides a home for a few bacteria. Eczematous skin always supports a relatively high population of bacteria, including potentially harmful varieties. *Staphylococcus aureus* is almost invariably present, but probably does little harm until its numbers reach a certain level. Examination by swabbing and culture, however, tells us only if they are present, not in what number, and is therefore a relatively uninformative exercise. There are ways of doing more accurate counts of bacteria on the skin but these techniques are not widely available. The only real value in taking ordinary swabs is to determine the sensitivity of the bacteria to antibiotics. Antibiotics can be put on to the plates and their effect on the growth of colonies studied. This helps the doctor to know if a particular infection will be susceptible to the antibiotic which he wants to use.

Occasionally, bacteria other than *Staphylococcus aureus* are responsible for infections in eczematous skin, and swabs can give the clue that this is the case. Once again, one has to be cautious about the interpretation of results, but it is important to try to identify the responsible bacteria in any infection that does not respond to initial treatment, because a change of medication may be necessary.

We can now reach some conclusions regarding the role of bacteria in atopic eczema. Firstly, that large numbers of potentially harmful bacteria frequently colonise eczematous skin. Secondly, that these bacteria can exacerbate the eczema without any overt signs of infection. Thirdly, that bacterial infections, whether obvious or not, are a frequent cause of deterioration of the eczema. Fourthly, that the great majority of infections are caused by a particular variety of bacterium known as *Staphylococcus aureus*. And, finally, that 'taking swabs' does not tell one whether infection is present or not. A logical approach to the use of antibacterial treatment must be based on a clear understanding of these principles.

Antibiotics

The 'systemic' (internal) use of antibiotics in eczema is generally reserved for obvious and extensive infections, or for exacerbations in which one strongly suspects that infection is responsible. The first choice is generally erythromycin (Erythrocin, Erythroped). Erythromycin is safe, cheap and effective in the great majority of infections in eczematous skin. Other antibiotics are often used instead, particularly phenoxymethylpenicillin (Crystapen V, Distaquaine V-K, V-Cil-K), ampicillin (Penbritin), amoxycillin (Amoxil), cloxacillin (Orbenin), flucloxacillin (Floxapen), cefaclor (Distaclor), cephalexin (Ceporex), sodium fusidate (Fucidin), co-trimoxazole (Septrin, Bactrim) and trimethoprim (Monotrim, Ipral). Although each of these may be more suitable individually for other types of infection, none are generally superior to erythromycin in the treatment of infected eczema. Cloxacillin (Orbenin), flucloxacillin (Floxapen) and sodium fusidate (Fucidin) differ from erythromycin in being lethal to a smaller range of bacterial species; they have in medical terms a 'narrower spectrum of activity'. Although in all three instances this includes the important *Staphylococcus aureus*, other species of bacteria often accompany this one, and need to be treated in their own right. On the other hand, in a small minority of cases *Staphylococcus aureus* may be resistant to erythromycin and, in these circumstances, one of these three may be needed to treat the infection effectively.

'Resistance' tends to develop in bacteria if they are exposed for any length of time to amounts of an antibiotic less than that required to kill them, and it can be passed on from one type of bacterium to another. No antibiotic is lethal to all types of bacteria and some will survive treatment. Our intestines are full of bacteria that help digestion, and which we need to remain healthy. If a systemic antibiotic is used to treat an infection in the skin many of these gut bacteria will survive. Some of them will develop resistance to the antibiotic used, and may pass it on to other potentially harmful types of bacteria. This is fortunately only temporary; after a period the resistance usually disappears unless the antibiotic is used again. The problem with resistant bacteria is a small one in the home, but can be quite a big problem in hospitals where antibiotics are used frequently. As patients are usually in close contact with one another, resistance can spread and this is one reason why children with infected eczema are often nursed in separate rooms away from other patients.

Antibiotics are always prescribed for a predetermined period, be it 5, 7, 10 or 14 days. Even though the infection for which they were given may seem to be effectively treated after two or three days, they should always be taken for the full period. This is to try to ensure that every last bacterium is killed before stopping treatment. If they are not all killed, the infection is likely to become re-established quickly and this time the bacteria may have acquired resistance, precisely because they survived the previous inadequate treatment. So always take antibiotics for the full period. Similarly, 'Take three times daily' means 'Take every eight hours'. With all antibiotics, success depends on the maintenance of adequate levels in the blood throughout the 24 hours of each day. The instruction: 'Take four times daily' means 'Take every six hours', and every effort should be made to give it as nearly as possible every six hours, even if this means waking your child to give a dose at midnight. If the blood level does fall below a critical level, it allows the bacteria to proliferate afresh and this delays successful treatment. It may also allow bacteria to become resistant during the period when the concentration is low, and this may prevent successful eradication of infection.

Antibiotics are often applied directly to the skin ('topically') as part of the treatment of eczema, rather than being given systemically. This has advantages and disadvantages. The main advantage is that the danger of any internal side effects is avoided. The main disadvantage is the difficulty of being sure that the bacteria are adequately exposed to the drug, both because they may be proliferating in sites not being treated, such as inside the nose, and because the concentration of the drug in the skin may not be adequately maintained throughout the 24 hours of the day. Both these factors have the additional effect of encouraging bacterial resistance to develop. For these reasons, the principles involved in the use of topical antibiotics are different. Firstly, they should be used for severe skin infections only if a systemic antibiotic is also used. Secondly, drugs used for serious internal infections such as lung or kidney infections should never be used on the skin. This limitation applies particularly to sodium fusidate (Fucidin) and gentamicin (Genticin). A further problem is that some antibiotics have a strong tendency to cause allergies when applied to the skin; this is especially true of penicillin and related drugs, so much so that they are never used in this way.

Some antibiotics which are either too toxic to be given internally or which are not absorbed into the body from the intestines, can nevertheless be used safely on the skin. Examples include neomycin (Nivemycin, Neocortef), clioquinol (Vioform and Vioform-hydrocortisone) and chlorquinaldol (Locoid C). Tetracycline may stain the teeth if used in children under 12, but it can be used safely topically (Terra-cortil, Trimovate, Terramycin, Achromycin).

The way that doctors use these topical antibiotics in eczema varies a great deal. Some reserve them for obvious infections, others use them more readily – even when infection is not clearly present.

There is some evidence that topical corticosteroids (see p. 52) work better in eczema if combined with a topical antibiotic, and this reflects the fact that infection is such a frequent complication of eczema, even when it is indiscernible.

The problem with using topical antibiotics continuously is that, in time, resistance will inevitably build up and the beneficial effects will be lost. The other is the danger, albeit a small one with the antibiotics I have listed, that an allergy may develop which will then have the opposite effect and actually aggravate the skin condition. For these reasons, it is probably wisest not to use any single antibiotic-containing preparation continuously for periods exceeding about eight weeks at a time. An application containing a different antibiotic, or one that contains no antibiotic at all, should then be substituted.

Antiseptics

Antiseptics are poisons which in appropriate concentrations kill both human cells and bacteria. Because they are poisonous they cannot be used internally. On the other hand, in suitably diluted form they may often be useful for direct application to the skin. Antiseptics have the following main uses in eczema: (1) Antiseptic solutions, paints or lotions for treatment of weeping eczema; (2) Antiseptic solutions for the prevention of infection; and (3) Antiseptic creams for treatment of carriers of *Staphylococcus aureus*

(1) *Antiseptic solutions, paints and lotions for treatment of weeping eczema*. When eczema weeps, creams and ointments are not the best form of treatment. The aim of treatment is to dry up and stop the exudation and, when this has been achieved, ointments and creams can be started again. The use of liquid preparations which will evaporate is frequently the best approach. There are several alternative liquids which can be used in this way, the most effective being those which contain antiseptics; probably best of all are dilute solutions of either potassium permanaganate or aluminium acetate (known in the USA as 'Burow's solution'). These are made up as required in warm water from either crystals or a concentrate. The ideal proportions are one part of potassium permanganate to 8000 parts of water and one part of aluminium acetate to 500 parts of water. The affected areas of the skin can either be immersed in the warm solution or it can be applied to the skin as a wet compress. Probably the best way of making such compresses at home is to use old nappies or towels. These are soaked in the freshly-made solution and then placed on the area to be treated. Every five minutes or so the compress should be removed, squeezed out and replenished with more of the warm solution. Which method is chosen will depend largely on the site to be

treated. A hand or foot will probably be most easily treated by immersion, whereas the cheeks could be treated only by the wet compress method. Each treatment should last 15-20 minutes and 2-4 treatments given each day. A minor problem with potassium permanaganate is that it stains the skin a brownish colour – and anything else that comes into contact with it.

A simpler but less effective approach to treatment of weeping areas of eczema is to apply one of the antiseptic dyes which you will probably remember from your own childhood. Alternatives are magenta paint (also known as Castellani's paint), brilliant green paint and crystal violet paint. These have the advantage that they are already made up at the appropriate strength and that they will keep well for long periods. Their disadvantage is that, because they contain alcohol or phenol as preservatives, they may sting when first applied. Furthermore, their bright colour tends to be rather unpopular because it gets everywhere. They are best applied on cotton wool balls, taking the paint up from a saucer into which a little has been poured. The method of tipping the bottle on to a cotton wool ball held into the open end is to be avoided because it inevitably contaminates the remaining contents of the bottle. Ready-made antiseptic lotions are available without preservative – for example, domiphen lotion and aluminium acetate lotion. These tend to be preferred to the paints, but they have a shelf life of only four weeks or so once opened which is a serious disadvantage. Domiphen lotion is not widely available at present and there may therefore be difficulty in getting it made up. These lotions are applied in exactly the same way as the paints and like them are best kept in the fridge.

Antiseptic Solutions for Prevention of Infection. The liberal application of antiseptics to the skin should reduce the numbers of colonising bacteria and might therefore be expected to diminish the number of infections. Unfortunately, there are two snags. Firstly, that the most effective antiseptics tend to be irritant at the necessary concentrations and, secondly, that application of such chemicals to large areas of skin is inevitably accompanied by some absorption through the skin into the bloodstream. Since these chemicals are by their nature toxic, this is potentially hazardous with long-term use. My own feeling is that this approach should be reserved for children who have had a run of infections and in whom these infections have continued to occur, and that it should always be confined to children over the age of two years in whom the degree of absorption will be less. The mild antiseptic Savlon is available in concentrated form known as 'hospital concentrate' in 10ml or 25ml sachets, or in one litre bottles. 25ml (about one dessert-spoonful) can be added to the bathwater, and this probably has the additional benefit of helping to reduce transmission of *Staphylococcus aureus* from the child with eczema to other members of the family and vice versa. Even when diluted, domestic antiseptics such as Dettol tend to be too irritant to use in this way.

(3) *Antiseptic creams for treatment of carriers of Staphylococcus aureus*. Many entirely healthy people carry *Staphylococcus aureus* on their skin and particularly in their noses. These bacteria cause no trouble to such 'carriers' but are a potential source of infection for eczematous children. Sometimes a child with eczema will get a run of infections. Treatment with systemic antibiotics seems to clear up the infection, only for it to recur immediately each course has ended. In such cases it may well be that the problem is another family member who is quite innocently carrying the responsible bacteria. This is one time where taking swabs for bacteriological culture is genuinely useful because it will detect such carriers. The problem can be solved easily by massaging a suitable antiseptic such as Naseptin cream into the nostrils four times daily for 10 days. Where a child's eczema has been complicated by two or three infections closely following one another, it is worth treating all other family members in this way simultaneously. Getting them all together to take swabs is in practice unnecessary.

Bandages

Many people reject out of hand the idea of bandaging up a child with eczema. They feel it must be unkind and that it will only make matters worse by making the skin hot and therefore even more itchy. Surely, they argue, there must be a better way of treating eczema these days. This kind of prejudice is a pity because bandages can undoubtedly be of great value, providing an extra dimension to treatment of children with more severe eczema.

Bandages may be used in two ways, either to provide protection against scratching or as a vehicle for medications. Let us consider these separately.

Bandages for protection. Ordinary crepe bandages may be used for this purpose, but tubular bandages are far better. A good range of tubular bandages is produced by Seton Products; Tubiton, Tubinette and Tubigauz are all suitable. Tubigauz is all cotton; Tubinette is all rayon; and Tubiton is a mixture of the two. These are made in eight standard sizes:

- 00 – small fingers and toes
- 01 – larger fingers and toes
- 02 – bandaged fingers and toes (for example, over paste bandages)
- 34 – younger child's legs and arms
- 56 – older child's legs and arms
- 78 – younger child's head, baby's body
- T1 – younger child's body, older child's head
- T2 – older child's body.

These bandages are most often used to make mitts, and there is hardly a child with eczema for whom this is not useful. During the day a child's hands should be free for activity but at night mitts help to diminish the damage that can be done by scratching, without being too constraining. *The technique for making mitts* is illustrated in Figs 7.2, 7.3 and 7.4. Some mothers prefer to make mitts themselves from cotton material. This is done by cutting out hand-shaped pieces of material and sewing two together around the outside. These can be made double thickness by making a second slightly larger mitt, turning this one inside out so that the seam is hidden, and putting the smaller mitt inside. If a strip of material is sewn to the outside, this can be used to attach it to pyjamas at the wrist with a safety pin. Another piece of material or ribbon can be sewn on to the wrist of the pyjama sleeve and this can then be attached to the one on the mitt by tying a bow. Older children may prefer lightweight washable cotton gloves, which are also made by Seton Products. Whole arms and legs can be bandaged, the problem being to secure the end where the limb meets the body. One solution is to apply a stocking to the body itself, then to tie the arm or leg bandage to it; this technique is illustrated in Figs 7.5 to 7.10. Some parents bandage their children from head to toe before they go to bed each night and, though I certainly wouldn't recommend this for every child with eczema, all parents should ask themselves if more limited forms of bandaging could help their child.

Medicated bandages A wide range of such bandages is available. Most of them are impregnated with a paste and are made primarily for the treatment of leg ulcers in adults. It turns out that they can also be useful for treating eczema in children. I consider them to be very underrated. The most useful of all are those impregnated with either coal tar paste (Tarband or Coltapaste) or ichthammol paste (Ichthopaste of Icthaband). They are particularly helpful when lichenification (p. 21) is prominent. Unfortunately, some children cannot tolerate coal tar and their skin will appear to be 'burnt' by bandages which contain it. Such bandages are usually best avoided where there are extensive raw areas.

Those bandages which contain the fossil fish tar ichthammol (p. 58) are much milder and will generally be tolerated when coal tar bandages are not. On the other hand, their benefit is not as great, so wherever possible the coal tar bandages are preferable. Quinaband contains the antibiotic clioquinol, and can be helpful for infected eczema. Calaband is a mild paste bandage containing Calamine, ideal for inflamed, angry eczema.

All these bandages have a refreshing cooling effect when first applied. They can be successful in relieving irritation and also have healing properties, particularly those containing tar. Unfortunately, they are quite messy to apply. Another bandage is needed to cover the wet paste bandage. Some people use ordinary crepe bandages for this purpose, but these are not really ideal. I find that a rather special bandage called 'Coban' is best. This is an elasticated bandage which is self-gripping without incorporating any adhesive. It is pink and light, allowing air to pass through easily but providing some resistance to seepage of the paste. It is a great shame that this unique bandage is expensive and currently not prescribable; parents must therefore buy it from the chemist themselves, or obtain supplies directly from a helpful hospital supplies department. These bandages can be easily applied only to hands, arms, feet and legs. Most children find them surprisingly comfortable and, although they are generally most suitable for use at night, they may also be worn during the day because the Coban allows considerable freedom of movement. It seems best not to leave individual bandages on for more than 24 hours, though I have known cases where they have been successfully left on for three days at a time. Some mothers manage to eke out their

---

Opposite:

How to make night mitts out of tubular bandage. Cut off an appropriate length of bandage. Remember that it will need to be double the distance from the tip of the thumb to the wrist. The bandage is then slipped on so that it reaches the wrist at one end; the same length should still be hanging free at the other end. Now twist the bandage just beyond the end of the thumbnail, with the other fingers bent (Fig 7.2). The far end can now be pushed back over the hand, providing a double thickness. A fold containing both layers should be pinched up at the wrist, and then wrapped around the wrist to take up the slack (Fig 7.3); this fold should be taped down using micropore or any suitable adhesive tape (Fig 7.4).

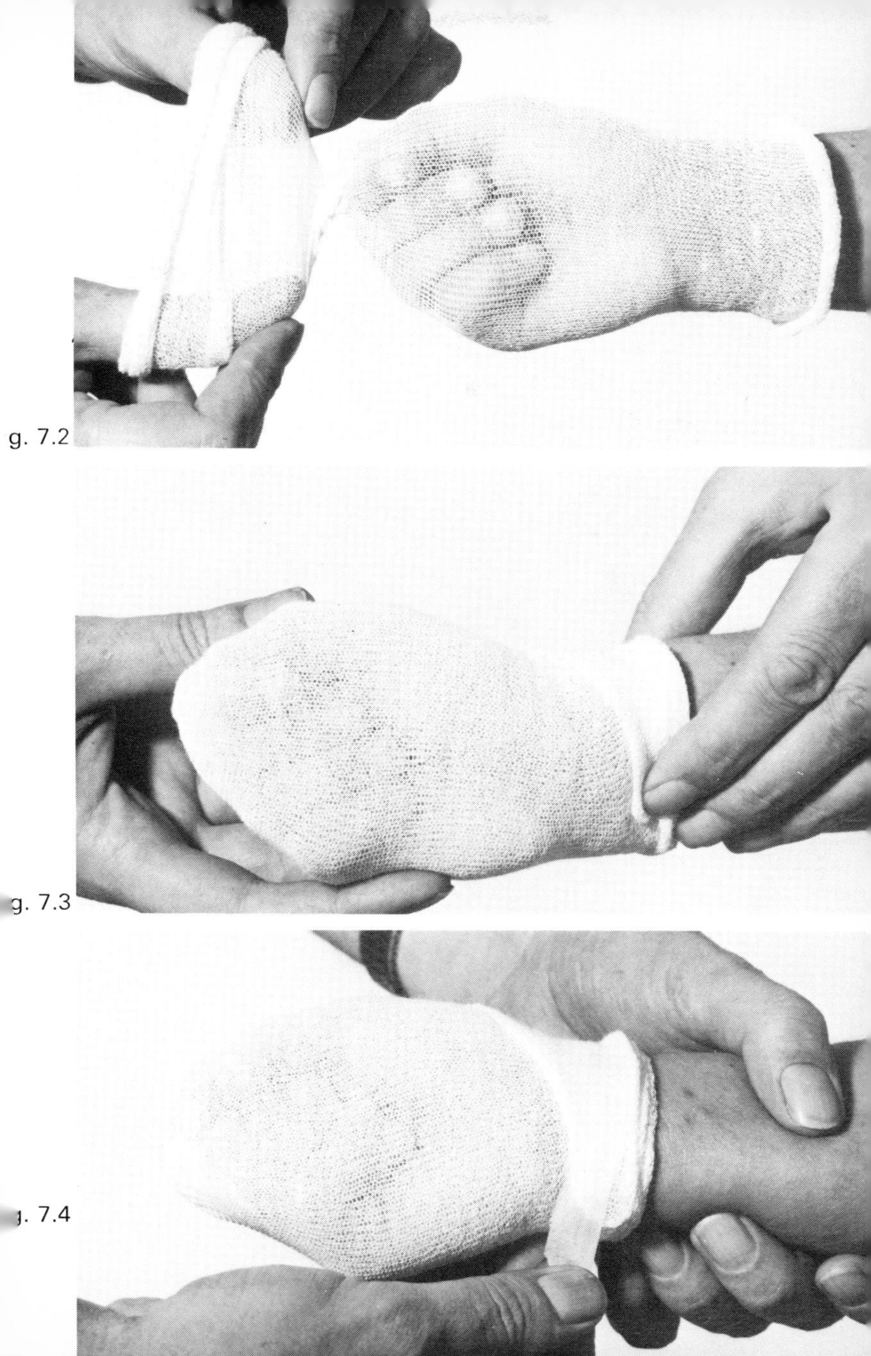
g. 7.2
g. 7.3
ı. 7.4

How to apply tubular bandage to an arm. Ideally a bandage is worn on the trunk to secure the tubular bandage on the arm. First, cut off a suitable length of bandage for the trunk. Cut a notch in both sides for the arms (Fig 7.5), then put on the bandage just like a T-shirt (Figs 7.6 and 7.7). Now cut off a suitable length of bandage for the arm. Allow a little extra to fold under at the wrist (Fig 7.8). At the top end, the bandage is secured to the trunk stocking by ties which are cut into the top of the arm bandage (Fig 7.9). Small holes are cut into the trunk stocking, and the ties passed through and knotted (Fig 7.10).

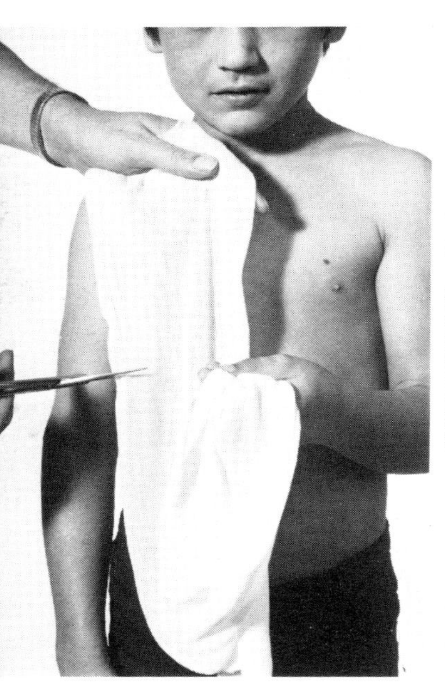

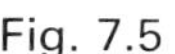

Fig. 7.5

Fig. 7.6

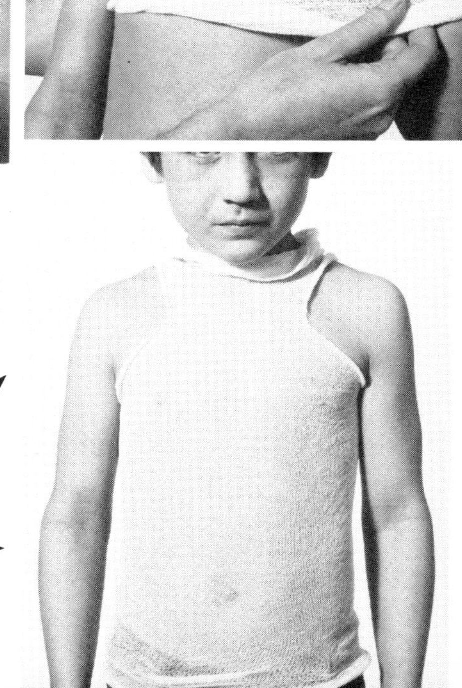

Fig. 7.7

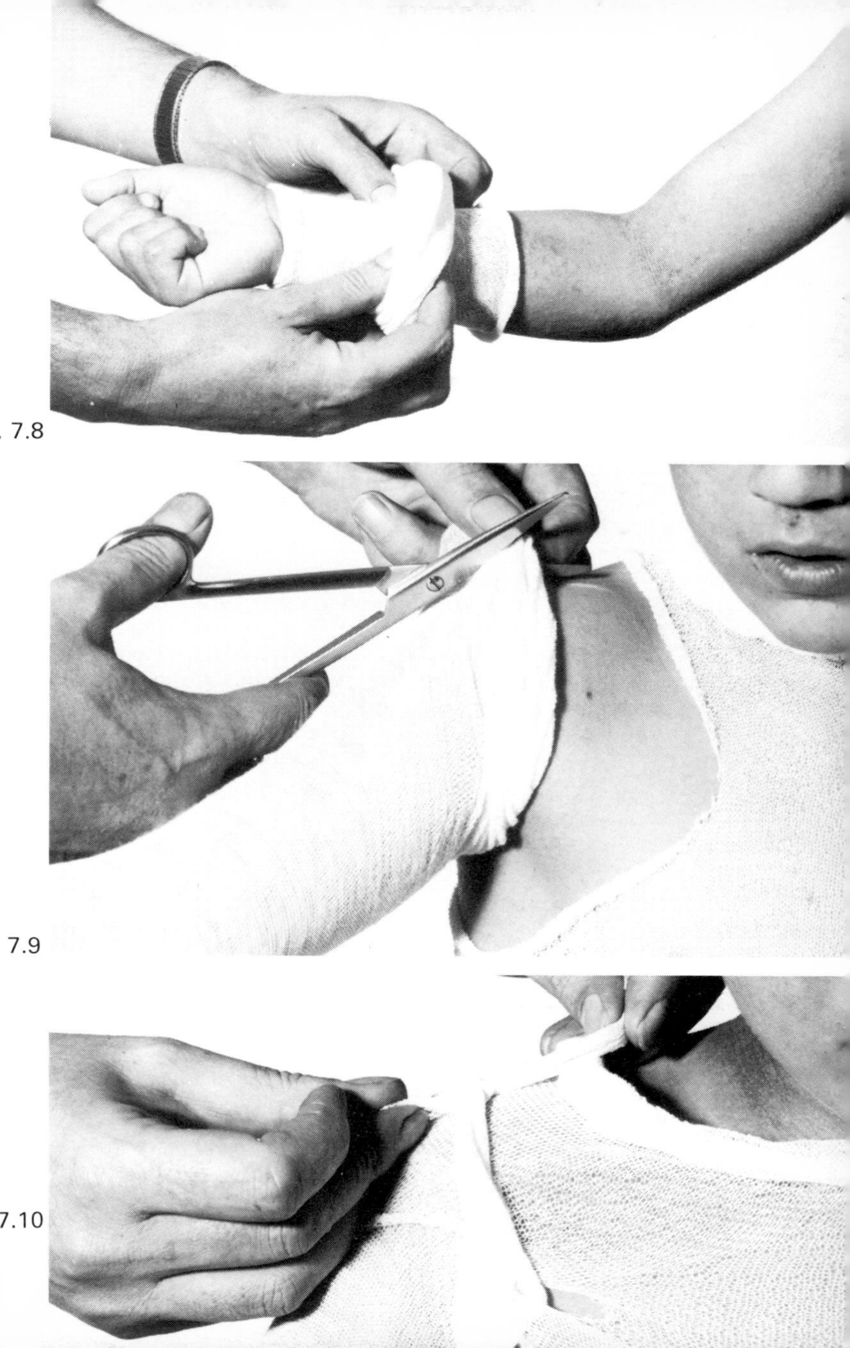

7.8

7.9

7.10

supplies by reusing or even washing the Coban once or twice. After washing, the elasticity tends to disappear. Paste bandage treatment is probably ideally used as a temporary measure from time to time, and this is how most parents seem to end up using them. The application of these bandages is illustrated in (i) the hand 7.11–14, (ii) the arm 7.15–18, and (iii) the leg 7.19–24.

How to apply paste bandages. The best time to apply a paste bandage is after the bath, when the skin is clean. The paste bandage should be applied fairly loosely as it will shrink slightly after a few hours.

The hand. Start at the wrist, and then come straight across the back of the hand to the little finger (Fig 7.11). Wrap the bandage around the little finger, and then cut it. Now, start again at the wrist and bandage the ring finger in exactly the same way. Then carry on to the other fingers, always starting at the wrist and cutting the bandage after wrapping up the finger (Fig 7.12). When you have finished, the back of the hand will be covered (Fig. 7.13), but the palm, which is rarely affected by eczema, will be left free (Fig 7.14), keeping the hand more comfortable.

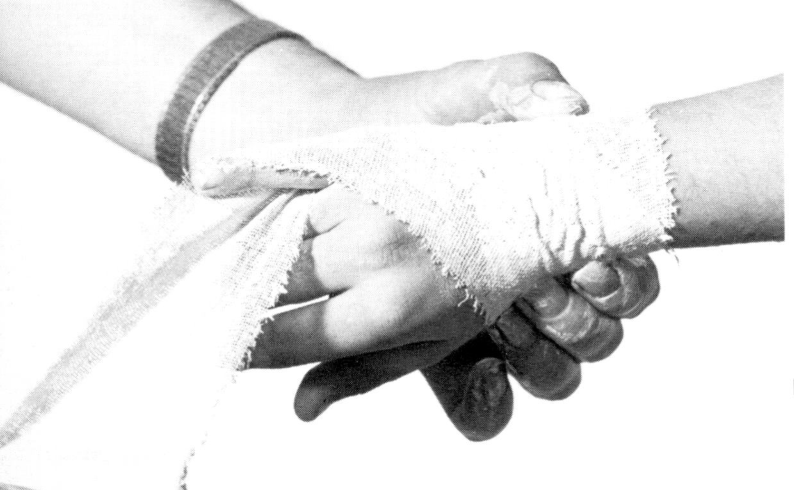

Fig.

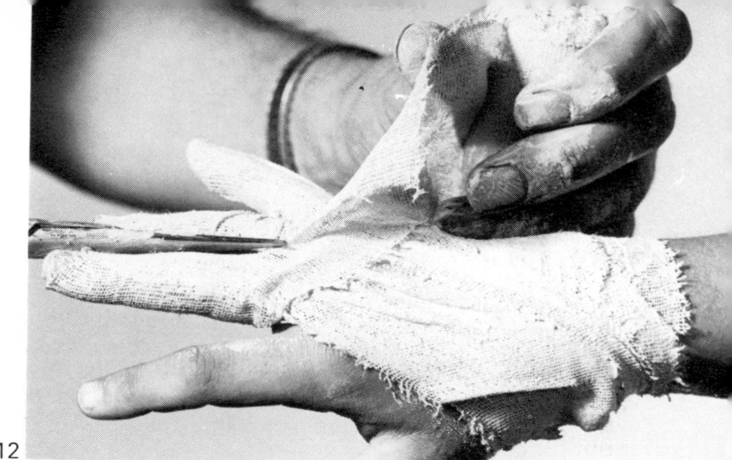
Fig. 7.12

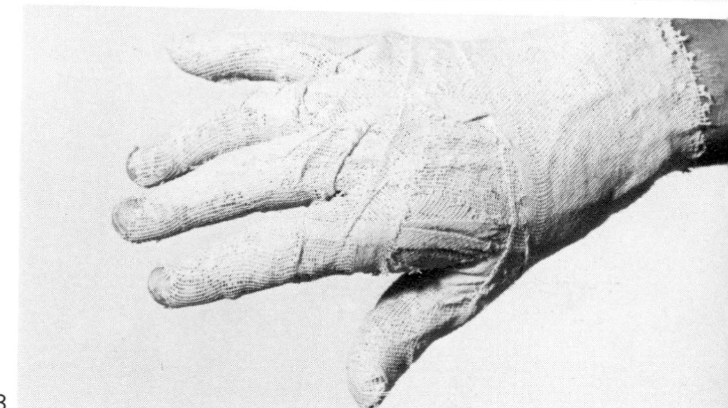
Fig. 7.13

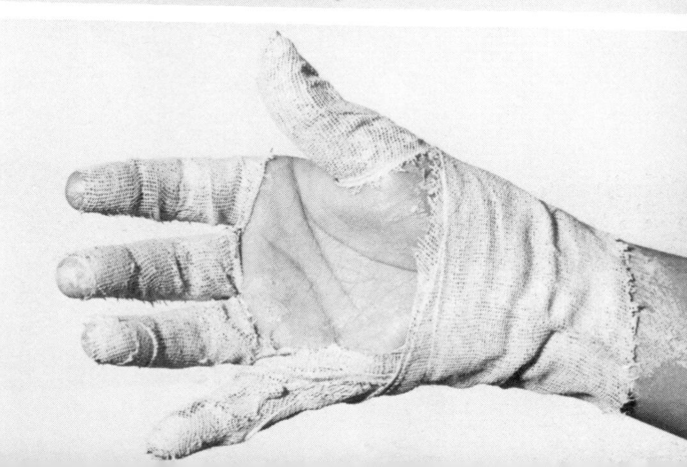
Fig. 7.14

The arm. Start at the wrist (Fig 7.15), and then work up the arm to the elbow (Fig 7.16). The elbow should be slightly bent. Reverse the direction of winding (Fig 7.17); this enables the bandage to slip slightly when in place, giving mobility at the elbow. It also helps to compensate for any shrinkage of the bandage. Now continue up the rest of the arm (Fig 7.18).

Fig. 7.15

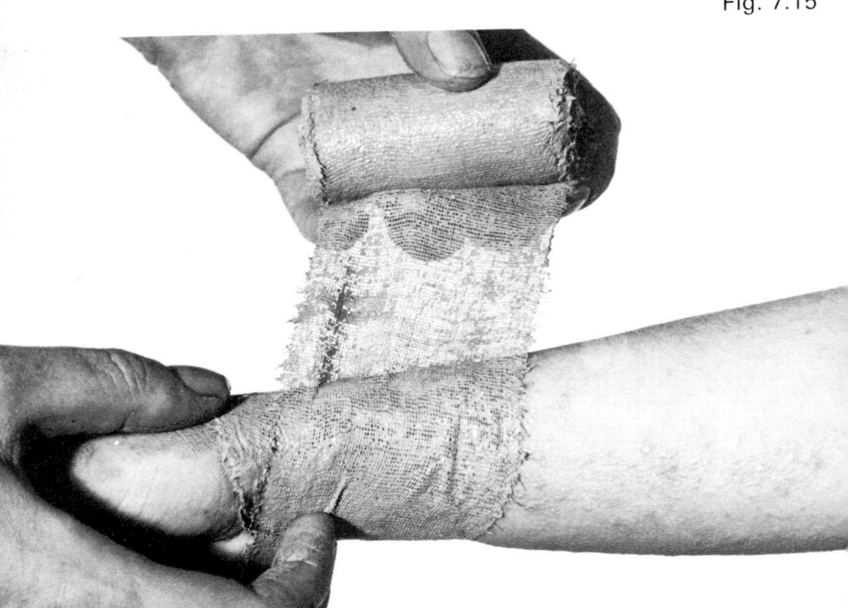

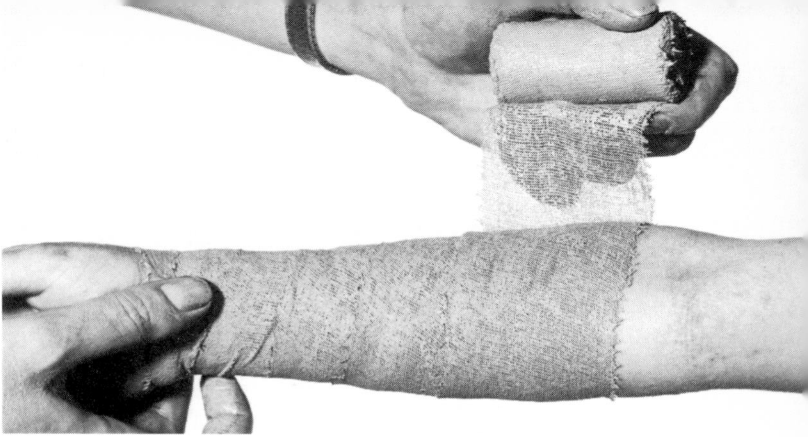

7.16

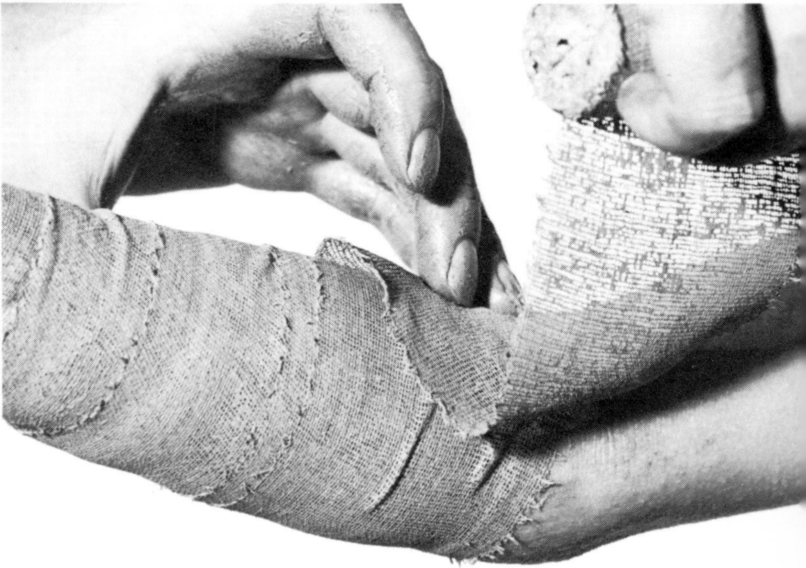

7.17

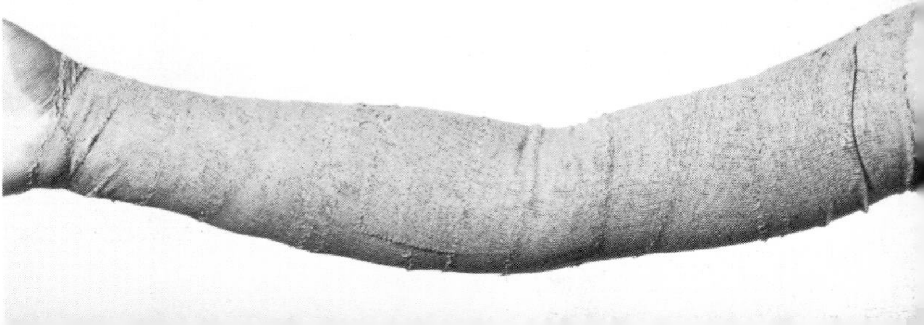

7.18

The leg. Start at the foot, which is best bandaged quite separately from the rest of the leg (Fig 7.19). Now bandage the ankle, again separately (Fig 7.20). Cutting the bandage avoids kinks, gives mobility at the ankle, and compensates for shrinkage by allowing the bandage to slip a little. Now bandage up the leg, occasionally reversing the direction of the winding to allow some slipping (Figs 7.21 – 7.22). Now apply the Coban, overlapping the paste bandage slightly at the ends. Wind it on with a little, but not excessive, stretch (Figs 7.23 and 7.24). Although it does grip itself, it nevertheless needs securing at the end with tape or a safety pin.

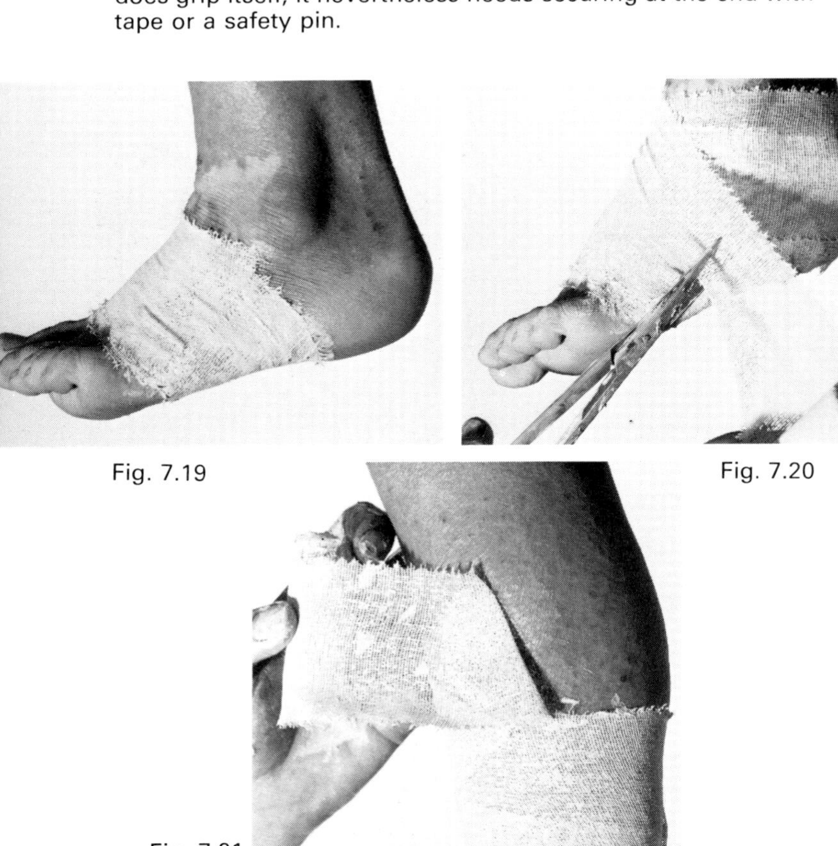

Fig. 7.19

Fig. 7.20

Fig. 7.21

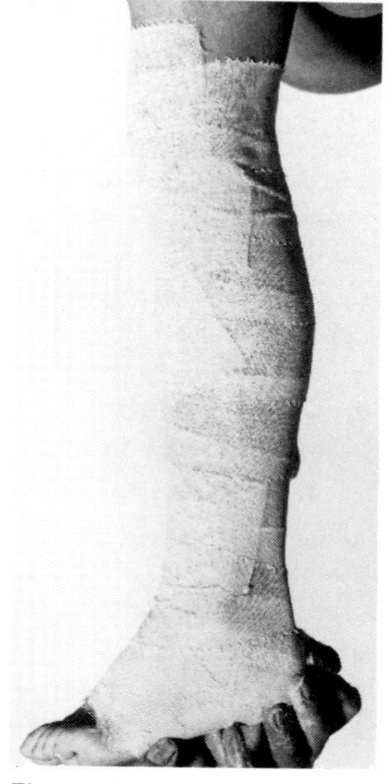

Fig. 7.22

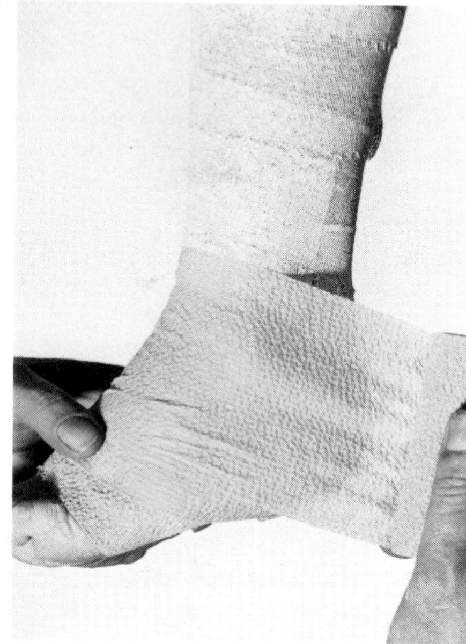

Fig. 7.23

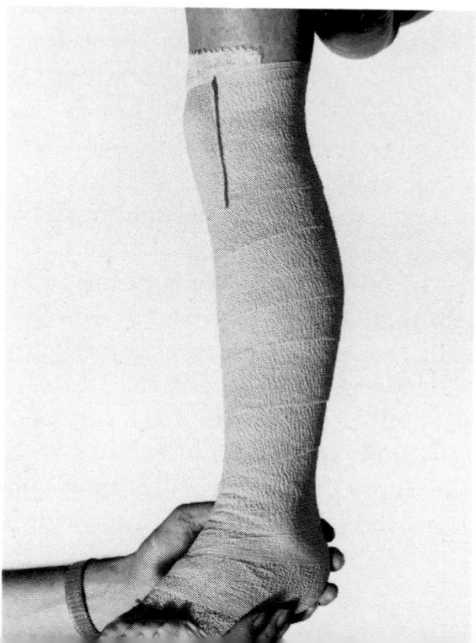

Fig. 7.24

The Scalp

The scalp is frequently affected by eczema, but is a difficult area to treat because the hair gets in the way. Fortunately, scalp eczema is often very mild and in such cases may require no more than a suitably medicated shampoo. Popular shampoos of this type include Polytar Liquid, Ionil T and Genisol. All these contain coal tar, but as mentioned earlier some individuals find this irritating. In these cases a non-tar shampoo such as Cetavlon PC is preferable.

A variety of preparations are now available where more intensive treatment of the scalp is necessary. In order to make treatment less messy, corticosteroids for scalp use are often made up in liquid form. These generally incorporate alcohol, which acts as a preservative and evaporates away after the liquid is applied. Such preparations include Locoid scalp lotion and Betnovate scalp application. Unfortunately, the alcohol may irritate eczematous scalps, and these preparations are perhaps not ideal in this condition. The Betnovate scalp application is in any case too potent for long-term use in children. Locoid scalp lotion is somewhat less potent and more suitable for use in children, though even this should probably be avoided in children under five years. The scalp is an area of skin through which absorption is particularly high. Synalar gel is an alternative non-greasy preparation, but is more difficult to apply to extensive areas of scalp and is also far too potent for prolonged use in children. One per cent hydrocortisone lotion (Efcortelan) is the safest corticosteroid preparation suitable for scalp use, and it does not contain alcohol.

Personally, I find corticosteroids rather unhelpful in scalp eczema generally and other approaches more useful. Salicylic acid is a traditional dermatological remedy for scaling disorders and is especially useful for the scalp. As for eczema treatment generally, ointments are superior, though their greasiness can cause special problems in the scalp. The best approach is to apply emulsifying ointment containing about 2% salicylic acid and to wash the hair out the following morning. The application process is time-consuming and fairly tedious. For the best results the hair should be parted and the ointment rubbed into the scalp where it is exposed along the parting. Further partings should then be made progressively across the scalp. Salicyclic acid, like anything else applied to the skin, will be absorbed into the blood. The amounts absorbed are not a problem except in babies, and this type of treatment is probably best reserved for those over two years.

Even more effective in severe cases is the combination of salicyclic acid and coal tar. The most popular formulation is known as compound coconut ointment (Ung. Cocois Co.), as the base contains natural coconut oil. Coconut oil has a melting point very close to body temperature, which means that it is fairly solid when applied, and turns to liquid once on the skin. This helps to spread the ointment in the scalp, the active ingredients being the tar and the salicylic acid. As always with tar, an irritant effect may preclude its use in certain individuals. This preparation is messy, but even so can be helpful enough to be worthwhile. It is applied in exactly the same way as the plain salicylic acid ointment.

For really intensive treatment, Ung. Cocois Co. may be applied at night, washed out every morning, and a corticosteroid such as Efcortelan lotion or Locoid scalp lotion applied after drying the hair.

Antihistamines

The itch of eczema results from the release of chemicals into the skin during the inflammatory reaction (see p. 18). Unfortunately, it is unclear exactly which of the many chemicals that may be released is actually responsible. At one time it was thought likely that it was a substance known as histamine. Drugs which could counter the effects of histamine ('antihistamines') were therefore tried out in eczema. Although they are undoubtedly helpful, they do not abolish more than a proportion of the itch, probably because substances other than histamine are also important. In adults, antihistamines almost invariably causes appreciable drowsiness, so much so that they are commonly used to help patients to sleep. This effect is rather less predictable in children. Drowsiness can cause problems during the day, such as irritability, lack of attention at school, and a slowing of reactions which can be potentially dangerous when cycling or crossing roads. For this reason, antihistamines are probably best avoided during the day except in special circumstances – for example, when a child is in bed or in hospital. On the other hand, this side effect may be turned to advantage when antihistamines are used at night – unless it persists the following morning.

A wide variety of antihistamines are available, among the most frequently prescribed being Vallergan, Phenergan and Piriton. Often relatively high doses are required to help eczematous children. These drugs should always be given by mouth, though some are available in creams. These are highly likely to cause allergy if applied to the skin over long periods and are therefore best avoided. The night-time dose should be increased until optimum effect is obtained, or until the degree of sedation becomes intolerable. A 'hangover' in the morning can often be avoided by giving it earlier in the evening. If not, the dose is probably too high and will require cutting back.

Antihistamines are not addictive, and when they are no longer needed their use can gradually be discontinued without problems, but it is often best to do this over a period. They are safe and have been used for many years in thousands of children without any significant long-term hazard coming to light.

It is often found that, with regular use, an antihistamine may appear to become less and less effective. The body seems to get used to it. This does not happen in every child. Up to a point, it can be overcome by an increase in dose but eventually, in some children, the antihistamine seems to have little effect at any dose and this is a sign that the drug should be stopped for a period. After an interval, the effect will usually be regained. Bearing this problem in mind, a case can be made for using these drugs intermittently during phases when the eczema is especially troublesome, and trying to have regular periods when they are not used. This helps to keep their effectiveness at a maximum for when they are most needed.

Some children just don't seem to get any benefit at all from antihistamines, and some even become rather hyperactive under their influence. In these cases they are best avoided. Unfortunately, other sedative drugs don't seem to be as helpful in eczema and children who get no benefit from antihistamines are rarely helped by these other drugs.

Treatment of the Underlying Allergies

Clearly, the most logical approach to the treatment of a child's eczema would be to identify its causes and then eliminate them. This is the way it would be done in an ideal world, but unfortunately we do not yet live in such a world. In the first place, we lack reliable tests to identify the responsible antigens and, in the second place, their complete avoidance would rarely be feasible.

My own feeling is that when a child's eczema is fairly mild it is best to stick with simple treatments such as moisturisers and topical corticosteroids. Only when this approach fails are the difficulties of allergy diagnosis and antigen avoidance really justifiable. When a child's eczema is severe, however, the effort is certainly worth while.

As we have already discussed in Chapter 4, the antigens that provoke atopic eczema tend not to be unusual things like drugs or lobster; they are almost always very ordinary things that surround us in our daily lives. They are everyday foods like eggs and milk, and environmental antigens like house dust mites, pollen and dander from our pets. And, to make matters even more complicated, it is not usually a question of allergy to just one of these things but to several and in some cases virtually all of them.

So how does one start to unravel all this? We have already considered the value of allergy tests in Chapter 2 and I will return to the subject again later. On skin testing, children with eczema generally react to a variety of common substances of the kind we have just mentioned. Unfortunately, so also do many other children who do not have eczema or any other problem (maybe as many as a third of all children), though many of them will undoubtedly develop eczema, asthma or hayfever later on. These skin tests do give clues, but clues that need careful interpretation if they are to be of any use. What is certain is that a blind belief that the results of skin testing can precisely identify the causes of a child's eczema will almost always lead to failure in treatment. One needs to seek other evidence that particular antigens are provoking a child's eczema. In practice, the best way to do this is to study the effect of avoidance, and to confirm any apparent benefit from avoidance by observing the consequences of reintroduction. A snag is that avoidance may not result in obvious improvement in a child's eczema unless *all* the principal causes are eliminated at once. This situation is somewhat analogous to that of a combination lock. Getting one number right is simply not good enough. In eczema, however, one can achieve much without getting *every* number right; a good proportion will usually do.

The best place to start is with foods. A child's food intake can be manipulated relatively easily, and, in many cases, food allergies do seem to be the major problem.

Food Allergy and Elimination Diets

The main problem one has in identifying foods that may be provoking a child's eczema is that virtually any food may be implicated. Parents sometimes ask me questions like: 'Do tomatoes cause eczema?' This is the wrong question. The right question is: 'Are tomatoes one of the things that cause *my* child's eczema?' Some foods do appear particularly likely to aggravate eczema, but almost any food can do so. The important thing is to identify those foods that are responsible in the individual case.

Another problem is that foods can aggravate eczema by

mechanisms other than allergy. As it happens, tomatoes often do this. Parents frequently notice that tomatoes make the area around the child's mouth red; other foods that tend to do this are oranges and Marmite. Such children may be truly allergic to these foods, but the redness is more often simply a consequence of direct irritation due to the acidity of tomatoes and oranges, or the saltiness of the Marmite.

In some children certain foods may cause a more intense reaction than just redness when they come into direct contact with the skin. Most characteristically this will take the form of weals at the site of contact, usually on the face but often on the fingers and hands as well. This reaction is known in medical language as 'contact urticaria'. It is due to a genuine allergy to the responsible food. It is, however, not the same thing as eczema and, just as in the case of the irritant reaction we have just discussed, the responsible food may cause no problem at all once swallowed. Contact urticaria occurs when the skin contains large amounts of IgE antibodies (see p. 8), and is exactly the same reaction that is elicited in the prick test (p. 8), but so vigorous that the skin does not even have to be broken to introduce the antigen. If the skin in contact with the antigen is already broken – as it frequently will be in children who have eczema – the reaction will be even more intense. Although foods that provoke contact urticaria will not necessarily cause any problem once swallowed, they nevertheless often do. Sometimes this provokes more generalised wealing (urticaria), usually within a few minutes. In other cases they may instead aggravate the child's eczema, something that will usually happen much more insidiously. Some children will experience a combination of all of these reactions.

On the other hand, food probably more often provokes eczema without also causing irritant reactions, contact urticaria or generalised urticaria. There is usually a delay between eating the food and worsening of the eczema, a delay which may vary from a few minutes to many hours. Often the first thing that happens is a vague widespread blotchy redness of the skin together with increasing itchiness. Following on from this redness, crops of tiny vesicles may start to appear (p. 19). Such a reaction would be a relatively violent one; more characteristically, the whole affair is much subtler, and the eczema simply gets a little worse in the areas already affected, the worsening starting almost imperceptibly after a delay of an hour or two. Because the foods that can provoke such reactions tend to be ones that are eaten several times each day and, because there may be many foods that can do this, the link between the eczema and the foods is only very rarely an obvious one. The severity of the eczema seems to fluctuate from hour to hour and from day to day, without any clear explanation. This lack of an overt cause-and-effect relationship between foods and eczema is one of the main reasons that so many people, medical and otherwise, find it difficult to accept that there is a relationship at all. Nevertheless, we do now have fairly strong evidence that foods *are* a major cause of eczema.

Although almost any food appears able to provoke eczema, two stand out from the crowd because of their particular propensity to do so; they are eggs and milk. The only really reliable way to exclude the possibility that eggs and milk are aggravating a child's eczema is by a trial period of complete avoidance. Unfortunately, these two foods are often important elements in children's diets, especially in the case of small children, and their elimination may result in serious nutritional deficiency if proper compensatory adjustments are not made. For this reason, elimination diets should never be attempted without the assistance of a trained dietitian. It must always be borne in mind that dietary treatment can have serious side effects, just like drug treatment. Dieticians are available in most hospitals, and general practitioners can put patients in contact with them, or this can be done through hospital specialists. Having given this warning, it will usually be found that diets free of egg or milk are quite straightforward and manageable. The protein lost from the diet may be replaced by eating more meat or by using a milk substitute, such as soya milk or goat's milk. Apart from supplying protein, the most important function of milk in children is to provide calcium, essential for normal growth of bones and teeth. This calcium must also be replaced, and many soya milks and goat's milk will do so, so long as at least half a pint (10 oz or 300 ml) is taken daily. Soya milks are nutritious and reasonably tasty, even if they take a little getting used to. Their main problem is their rather off-putting smell. This can be overcome to a great extent if they are taken from a bottle or a trainer cup, rather than from an open cup. While children are still drinking in this way, they will generally accept soya milk perfectly happily. Acceptance becomes more of a problem when they are older than this, and this is when goat's milk may come in useful.

It has been known for many years that milk must be 'modified' for safe use in babies under six months. 'Unmodified' milk can be dangerous and can, for example, cause fits. 'Modification' is a process by which the balance of proteins, fats, carbohydrates and salts is altered to resemble more closely that found in human milk. All cow's milk-based baby milks are now treated in this way, but this is not yet true of all the available varieties of soya milk. Fortunately there are now five suitably 'modified' soya milks, all widely available, principally through chemists; they are Formula S (Cow and Gate), Wysoy (Wyeth), New Velactin (Wander), Granolac (Granose) and Prosobee (Mead Johnson) (Fig 7.25). The last of these is available only on prescription, reflecting the manufacturer's

Fig. 7.25 Soya 'milks' available in the UK which are suitably modified for infant feeding. All contain added calcium, and all are good substitutes for cows' milk at any age.

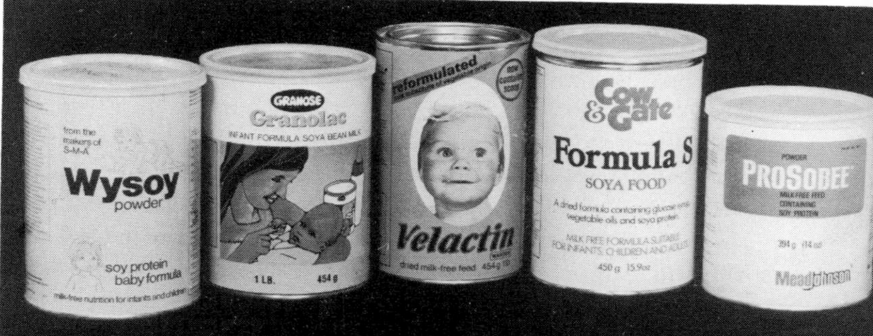

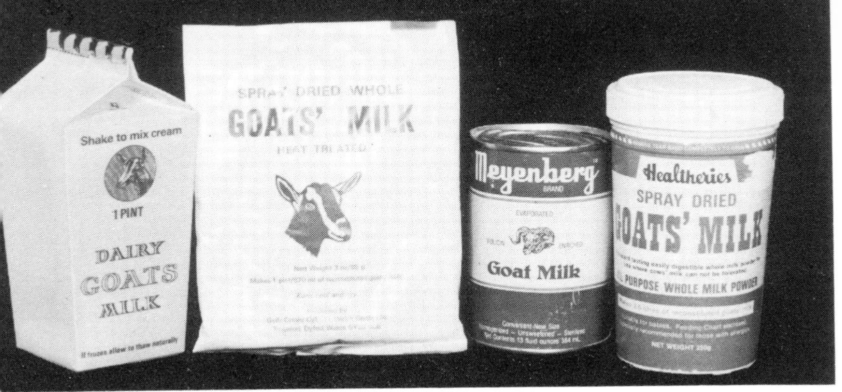

Fig 7.26 Examples of goat's milk, as it can be purchased in the UK. None of these are suitable for feeding to small babies, and only the heat-treated forms are really safe for small children.

belief that such preparations should be used only on medical advice.

There are four main snags to consider with goat's milk. The first is availability. A reliable supply of good quality goat's milk may be difficult to find, though this has become distinctly easier than in the past. At present, goat's milk is generally available in either liquid form or frozen (Fig 7.26). In rural areas it can often be obtained direct from a producer. In towns it is often stocked by health food shops and is even distributed by some supermarket chains, notably Safeway. The high turnover in such a supermarket does ensure that the product is likely to be both fresh and relatively inexpensive, and I would for these reasons particularly recommend this source. With frozen goat's milk, the condition of the milk may be uncertain, and I would tend to be cautious about buying it in this form. On the other hand, goat's milk does freeze well and it is quite a good idea to buy a largish stock of fresh liquid milk and freeze it oneself as quickly as possible in the rapid-freeze part of one's own freezer. Goat's milk is also fed to baby goats (hardly surprising!), which means that it can be difficult to find during the kidding season. Freezing down a small store is the best way to avoid this problem. Dried goat's milk will probably soon become available, which should solve many problems.

The second snag is a more serious one. Strict controls are enforced to ensure the freedom of dairy cattle from certain dangerous infections, such as tuberculosis and brucellosis, which are transmissible in milk. No such controls exist in the case of dairy goats, though these infections are in fact rare in British goats. In addition, the milking sheds of dairy cattle farms are regularly visited to check on hygiene and the milk itself is regularly tested to monitor its content of potentially harmful bacteria. Such bacteria get into the milk as a result of mastitis (infection of the udders), and by contamination from the cow's faeces and the farmer's hands. As a final precaution the milk is always pasteurized, a process in which it is heated for several minutes to a fairly high temperature, short of boiling. This sterilizes it, just as boiling would, but without diminishing its nutritional value or spoiling its flavour. Although I am certain that most goat's milk producers do maintain high standards of hygiene voluntarily, the goats are generally hand-milked – a method which itself increases the likelihood of contamination from the milker. Furthermore, the milk is generally unpasteurised. When we have ourselves checked the bacterial content of goat's milk obtained from various sources we have almost invariably found that it contains potentially harmful bacteria. For this reason it is wise to boil it, especially if it is to be given to children under two years of age, because pasteurization is not a practical proposition in the home. We recommend boiling for two minutes. The milk can then be cooled down and drunk cold. Unfortunately, the boiling does change the flavour for the worse and does reduce its content of some vitamins, especially folic acid which is already relatively low in goat's milk. Even so, most children will be getting an adequate supply if they eat fresh leafy green vegetables, kidneys or liver. Cooking only lowers the content of folic acid in these foods; it doesn't destroy it altogether. If a child eats little of these foods, supplementary folic acid should be given.

The third snag is that goat's milk is entirely unsuitable for babies under six months of age. Unboiled it is positively dangerous, as the bacteria it often contains may cause lethal infection in infants. But even boiled it is hazardous, because it is not 'modified'.

The fourth snag with goat's milk is that many of the proteins it contains are virtually indistinguishable from proteins in cow's milk. If children are allergic to one of these, the change to goat's milk may make little difference to their symptoms. This phenomenon can be illustrated by an experiment that has been done in guinea-pigs. Guinea-pigs can be made so allergic to cow's milk that 100 out of 100 allergic guinea-pigs will have serious reactions if later given cow's milk. When such guinea-pigs are instead given raw goat's milk 70 out of the 100 will have reactions. This is a measure of how similar the two milks actually are. If, on the other hand, the goat's milk is first boiled, the number of guinea-pigs having reactions falls from 70 to 30. This is because boiling considerably changes the properties of the proteins in the milk. This is a second good reason to boil goat's milk.

In my hospital we often ask children who are avoiding egg and milk to avoid chicken at the same time, because some of the proteins in chicken and egg are identical, as one might expect.

If an egg and milk free diet is going to help, it will usually do so within 4–6 weeks. The full benefit may not be seen if the diet is abandoned too early. If it proves helpful, the diet should probably be maintained unchanged for about one year, and the dietitian should check on your child's nutrition at least once during this time. At the end of the year, you will need to find out whether your child can now eat these foods without problems. This is best done by trying the eliminated foods again, one by one. Ideally, a full week should be set aside for each item. If this were milk, for example, a teaspoonful only should be given on the first day if there is any reason to believe that the allergy may be intense. If not, you can give a full glass of milk on this first day. If no adverse effects are apparent following this first dose, give between half and a full pint on each of the next six days. If at any time during the week you think that the eczema is becoming worse, stop the reintroduction. If you feel that there may have been an unrelated explanation for the deterioration you could try again later. If, at the end of the week, there has been no change in your child's eczema, you should have no worry about reintroducing milk into the diet on a more permanent basis. It is entirely wrong to expect to be able to tell whether your child reacts to a food by giving a small amount from time to time. It is often found that the food must be given in quite large amounts on successive days to unmask the allergy.

Parents often have strong suspicions that particular foods can aggravate their child's eczema. Apart from egg and milk themselves, the foods that are most often incriminated in this are nuts, tomatoes, fish and food colourings and preservatives. Where there is any reason to suspect any particular foods, they should also be avoided in the elimination diet in addition to egg and milk and chicken.

In fact, reactions to articifial colouring and preservatives in foods appear so common that it may be a good idea to include these in the elimination, even if one has no other reason to suspect them. After egg and milk, they seem to be the next most important dietary factors in eczema. They can largely be avoided by keeping to fresh foods, but to do the job thoroughly you again need help from a dietitian. Unfortunately, these additives are now very widely employed in the food industry. The use of preservatives is to some extent justifiable, since in their absence many foods would rapidly deteriorate. They are found in greatest amounts in prepared meats and sausages and, paradoxically, in virtually all liquid medicines. An undertaker I met recently commented that bodies seem to keep much longer nowadays; he wondered whether this could be because we all now eat so much preservative. There may be some truth in this. If there is any justification for the use of preservatives, there is none at all for the use of artificial colouring in foods. It seems to me that progressively more and more colour is added to food each year, and I have the distinct feeling that the problem is greater in Britain than in most other parts of Europe and North America. For example, orange squash seems to become more and more lurid each year, and some well-known brands of lollipop now stain the face indelibly for over 24 hours. The manufacturers claim that more brightly-coloured foods sell better. Take kippers as another example. The natural smoked kipper is a dull grey colour. Place a natural grey kipper and a bright yellow kipper side by side, and apparently the housewife will always choose the yellow one. Hens are fed a yellow dye to make the yolks of their eggs a deeper colour. The housewife apparently considers this bright yellow yolk to be a sign of a good egg. Surely it is time for us all to put on pressure to stop all this silliness? However, I mustn't get off the point. Colours do seem to be common provokers of eczema, especially the orange dye tartrazine and its chemical relatives.

Before going on, it might be a good idea to summarize what I have said so far about dietary treatment in atopic eczema. I hope it does not seem too confusing. Although some parents may have reason to believe that certain foods make their children's eczema worse, it is commoner for there to be no apparent link between foods and a child's eczema. This appears to be because the link is concealed, and it has in fact been shown in careful studies that as many as two out of every three children with eczema will benefit from a simple manipulation of the diet. In other words, dietary treatment is worth a try even if there seems to be no obvious link between foods and eczema in a particular child. Because there is no simple way of knowing which foods are relevant in the individual case, the best approach is simply to try elimination of those foods which have been found overall to be most frequently relevant. Those foods are eggs and milk, closely followed by colouring and preservatives. A diet avoiding these items is certainly worth trying if your child's eczema is not adequately controlled by ordinary treatments. It is, however, unwise to try this sort of diet without the advice of a trained dietitian, firstly because you may not succeed without help in completely eliminating these items and, secondly, because elimination diets can be hazardous if their effects on your child's nutrition are not carefully considered.

What is the next step if a simple diet such as this fails to provide any benefit in spite of being done perfectly? This could mean either of two things. It may be that foods simply aren't relevant in your particular child, or it may be that the relevant foods have not been identified. My own experience of treating children with diets suggests that the second explanation is more often, though not always, the correct one. There are one or two centres which specialise in taking the dietary approach a stage further. These centres each tend to adopt slightly different methods. One method which has been widely used is the so-called 'rotating' diet system. In this system all foods are divided up into groups – for example, dairy produce, cereals, meats etc – and each group of foods is individually excluded in rotation. One might therefore start off with a fortnight without dairy produce; then the dairy produce would be reintroduced and one would go on to a fortnight without cereals, until all groups had in their turn been eliminated. This type of approach would be fine if only one food, or one group of foods, were usually implicated. In other varieties of food allergy, such as urticaria, this is in fact often found to be the case, but in atopic eczema it only rarely appears to be so simple. Unfortunately, it is more usual for several, or even many, foods to play a part in causing atopic eczema, and therefore a different approach is needed, one which can identify a variety of causative foods simultaneously. The approach I personally favour may not turn out to be best, but it does fulfil this condition, and has been used successfully in quite a number of children.

After eggs, milk, colours and preservatives, all other food items seem more or less equally likely to provoke eczema. Therefore, if exclusion of these four has failed to produce the desired improvement, further guesswork is almost certainly doomed to failure because of the vast number of foods which may still be playing a role. The logical approach would be first to cut out *all* food for a week or so! This is, of course, entirely out of the question, and should never even be contemplated. Several centres around the world have tried to use 'space diets' as an alternative. These are complete liquid diets which contain all necessary nutrients in a predigested form to which one cannot be allergic. The trouble is that they taste fairly horrible, unless heavily disguised by flavourings, and flavourings are, of course, no good for these purposes. It may be possible to persuade an adult to live off this type of food for a few days, but children quite understandably will not usually have anything to do with it. One therefore has to compromise, and a reasonable approach is to use a regime that restricts the diet to a single meat, a single vegetable, a single carbohydrate and so on. Each individual constituent is selected because it has been found individually unlikely to be implicated in causing eczema. We have called these diets 'oligoallergenic' ('oligo' is the Greek for 'few'; 'allergen' is any antigen which can cause allergy). Here are two examples, in outline:

Oligo-allergenic diet 1
turkey
cabbage
potato and potato flour
stewed apple
Kosher (milk-free) Coffee-mate
Tomor (milk-free) margarine
White sugar and golden syrup
Vitamins and minerals

Oligo-allergenic diet 2
lamb
carrot
rice and rice flour
rhubarb
soya milk
Tomor (milk-free) margarine
White sugar and golden syrup
Vitamins and minerals

Just as with simpler diets, these should never be attempted without the help of a dietitian. We normally try one of these oligoallergenic diets for an initial period of no longer than three weeks. If this results in definite benefit, the next stage may be embarked on. The idea during this second stage is to reintroduce, one at a time, all those foods which were eliminated during the first stage. In this way, those which make the eczema worse may be individually identified. As you can imagine, this tends to be a slow, painstaking and difficult process, and for this reason this type of approach is only justified and worth while in the case of severely eczematous children. One new food is tried each week and it is given to the child in a normal serving on each day of that week. A full week is needed, because a single dose of a food may cause no adverse reaction, whereas several doses given regularly over a number of days will do so. If a food is eaten in this way on each of the seven days of the trial period without any worsening of the eczema (or any other harmful effect), it may subsequently be given freely at any time. If it does cause problems, it is once more eliminated from the diet. In the case of any doubt, the food is best eliminated again to be reintroduced once more later on. In this way, a list of foods that seem to provoke the child's eczema can gradually be built up, and at the same time the diet will (one hopes) be progressively expanded.

But what if the initial oligoallergenic period produces no real benefit? Once again, the explanation may be that foods are not the main problem, and the message may therefore be that one should look elsewhere for the main causes of the child's eczema. Nevertheless, an alternative explanation might be that the oligoallergenic diet itself contains something which can provoke eczema in that child. For this reason, it is often worth while trying a second and completely different oligoallergenic diet. If this still fails to do the trick, one is really forced for practical purposes to abandon this type of approach, whatever the reason for its failure.

I am often asked, 'How long is the interval between eating a food that provokes eczema and the resulting exacerbation?' Our studies have helped to cast some light on this question and it is clear that it can be highly variable. The exacerbation may be apparent within minutes, but often it is delayed but is probably not longer than 24 hours. The more often the food is given, the shorter the interval seems to become and, as I have already mentioned, a single dose may fail to produce any adverse effect where several doses over a period will do so. If a child has been avoiding milk, for example, one often finds that it is not until the third or fourth day of drinking half a pint daily that there is any deterioration in the eczema. In fact, it is commoner to find this pattern of response than one in which there is an immediate reaction on the first day. The question is whether the reaction on the third day is a reaction to the milk given on the second or third day. The other problem is that the reactions themselves may be very different in type in different children, though reactions to individual foods seem to be more or less uniform in any particular child. The most characteristic reactions are: increasing redness, usually widespread but sometimes just affecting the face, and/or a general increase in itchiness.

Non-food Allergy

Although foods appear to be of particular importance as causes of atopic eczema, a part is often played by allergies to things other than foods, and in some cases these may even constitute the main problem. The principal non-food allergens are characterised by their tendency to form airborne particles. These are the particles which can be seen in their millions in shafts of sunlight, though individually they are invisible. These particles are breathed in and are frequently implicated in the cause of asthma, sometimes in children who also have eczema but just as often in children who do not (see Chapter 9). People are often surprised to learn that only a minute proportion of the airborne particles we breathe in actually enters the lungs. Most of them stick to the moist walls of the nose, mouth and large air passages. The tubular passages which take air down to the lungs are provided with millions of microscopic hair-like projections which move together in such a way that the fluid on their surface is steadily wafted upwards towards the throat, and from there down into the stomach. The same cleansing mechanism is present on the internal lining of the nose, so that most of the airborne particles that are inhaled eventually pass down into the gut, just like food. The total amount of such particles inhaled each day may reach several grams. In other words, these airborne allergens differ from foods only in the way that they enter the body. After that, the two share much the same fate. Nevertheless, antigens may enter the blood from the particles caught on the linings of the air passages and the nose. It is possible that absorption of antigens by these routes is of great importance.

You will recall that I described how certain foods occasionally cause an allergic reaction when they come into direct contact with the skin (see page 87), a reaction known as contact urticaria. Airborne allergens can almost certainly have a similar effect. These airborne particles land on the skin the whole time. Where the skin is already affected by eczema, moistness will serve both to trap these particles and then to dissolve out the antigens (p. 8) which they contain. The skin surface barrier (p. 1) is impaired on eczematous areas and here these dissolved antigens will be able to pass through fairly freely. The itching this causes provokes more scratching and thus more damage. In its turn this both attracts more particles and further compromises the skin barrier. In this sort of way, airborne allergens may play an important role in many children with eczema in addition to any effects they may have following inhalation. Since this contact reaction is caused by IgE antibodies (see p. 8), skin tests using airborne allergens can help to give clues that this may be happening, and may also identify the likely provoking allergens.

In summary, certain airborne substances may possibly provoke eczema in exactly the same way as foods can, because the antigens they contain will enter the blood after they have been inhaled. These airborne antigens can also contribute to skin damage in eczema by contact with eczematous skin, by provoking a reaction of the contact urticaria type. Where this contact reaction is important, skin testing can be helpful, in contrast to its limited value in the case of food allergens.

Let us now consider individually the most allergenic varieties of airborne particles.

Pollens. Pollens consist of individual cells which are required for the fertilisation of seeds in plants. They are the plant equivalent of spermatozoa in animals. Pollen is transferred from plant to plant by either insects or the wind. Those plants which use insect pollination generally have brightly coloured flowers. They produce only small quantities of pollen, which is sticky and does not become airborne in significant quantities. For this reason, the pollens of flowering plants only rarely cause allergies. The pollen allergy problem is caused by the pollens of those plants which use the wind as their means of transport. Because this method is relatively inefficient, such plants produce vast quantities of pollen to ensure that some gets to the target. Generally these are plants of unimpressive appearance, and the species which are most important from the allergy point of view differ from country to country. In the United Kingdom, the major offenders are grass pollens, followed in importance by a variety of tree pollens. The production of pollen is a seasonal event. In the UK, grasses pollinate between the beginning of May and the end of July, and trees somewhat earlier – generally between the beginning of April and the end of May.

It can be difficult to establish whether pollen is an important provoker of eczema in the individual child. As I have mentioned, skin testing can give a helpful clue, but unless the test reaction is a very big one it certainly does not prove the case. The most suggestive feature of pollen allergy is its seasonal nature. Thus, if your child's eczema is regularly worse during May and June, you may be justifiably suspicious of grass pollen. In the case of the child who appears to be allergic to grass pollen, some simple precautions can help to reduce exposure, though it is clearly much more difficult to eliminate grass pollen than, say, a particular food. During the season, the allergic child should be kept indoors whenever grass or hay is being cut in the immediate neighbourhood. Windows should, as far as possible, be kept closed, both in the house and when travelling by car. The ultimate precaution is to install an electrostatic precipitator to remove pollen particles from the air entering the house. The entire air supply must enter the house through the precipitator, and windows must all be kept sealed to achieve the best results. Such machinery is quite popular in other countries, but is rarely used in the UK. The recently available table-top air filtering devices may possibly be helpful to some extent.

Eczema due to grass pollen allergy is at present the only type of eczema that appears likely to benefit from desensitisation injections. This type of treatment is worth considering if a child's eczema shows appropriate seasonal exacerbations, and when there is a strong response to a grass pollen skin test. The most common method of desensitisation treatment used in this country is to give a course of three injections in increasing strengths of a commercially available pollen extract, at weekly or fortnightly intervals. It is often found that each injection causes prompt but temporary exacerbation of the eczema. Far from being a reason to discontinue the treatment, this type of reaction seems to predict a favourable response to treatment. The problem with desensitisation treatment is the danger of more serious reactions and, although it is extremely unusual, children have died during treatment. This danger is minimised by careful supervision, but many doctors feel that the risks are too great to justify the treatment in all but exceptional cases.

House dust mites. As you can imagine, house dust contains a dreadful mixture of things. Although it has been known for many years that it can provoke allergies, exactly which of its constituents is responsible was until recently unknown. It has now become clear that the main culprit is the mite which goes by the name of *Dermatophagoides pteronyssinus*. This tiny creature is so small as to be effectively invisible, and literally millions live in the average home. Mites are closely related to spiders, and strictly-speaking are therefore not insects. The shed skin flakes from humans and domestic pets form an important element of their diet. Careful research has shown that it is their droppings which cause most of the allergy problem, and it is relevant that these droppings are very similar in size to pollen grains, having the same property of becoming airborne under the right conditions. House dust mites like environments where there is moisture, warmth and a good supply of food. Climatic factors seem to affect their population, and they are generally most numerous in the autumn from August to October. They like living in soft furnishings of all sorts, particularly carpets and mattresses. They are likely to be particularly populous where plenty of food is available. The immediate environment of the child with eczema is likely to suit them ideally from this point of view, and it has been shown that the mattresses and bedrooms of eczematous children contain mite populations many times greater than normal.

Unfortunately, it is even more difficult to establish whether the house dust mite is playing a role in provoking a child's eczema than it is in the case of grass pollen. The mite population remains fairly high throughout the year but, as I have mentioned, there is something of a 'mite season' in the autumn. You should therefore be suspicious of house dust mites if your child's eczema is regularly worse at this time of year. As in the case of grass pollen, a skin test may be helpful. A strongly positive test indicates at least that direct skin contact with the mite and its droppings could cause wealing and itching in eczematous areas. It should alert one to the possibility that inhaling the droppings could also make the child's eczema worse, though a negative test probably does not exclude this.

An attempt to reduce exposure to house dust mite allergens should be made wherever there is any reason to suspect it could be worsening a child's eczema. Because it can be so difficult to recognise this link, in my view it makes sense to undertake anti-mite measures in *any* household where there is a child with eczema. The more difficult the eczema is to control by other means, the more effort should be made to eradicate the house dust mite.

The following measures represent a sensible regime that is not too demanding. Let us first consider your child's bedroom. Ideally any child with eczema should have his or her own bedroom, and anti-mite efforts should be concentrated on this room. Carpets are particularly attractive to house dust mites, so linoleum or similar flooring is ideal. Gaps between skirtings and the floor should be eliminated. Dispense with rugs. The mattress and pillows should be enclosed in plastic covers. Although it might seem the best idea to enclose the mattress completely, I suspect that it is better to use a cover which leaves some space underneath through which the mattress can breathe a little. Pillows that are completely enclosed should be taken out regularly for airing; the same applies to mattresses that are fully enclosed. A good source of suitable plastic covers is Keys of Clacton Ltd, 132 Old Road, Clacton-on-Sea, Essex C015 3AJ, who operate a mail order business and are suppliers to many hospitals.

Duvets are a good idea, but choose a man-made filling, wash the duvet itself frequently – say weekly – and the sheets and pillowcases daily. If your child prefers blankets, choose acrilan or cotton ones because these are easier to wash and dry than woollen ones. Choose man-made washable fillings for pillows. Use plastic material for curtains rather than fabric. Chairs should be of painted wood or plastic and not upholstered. Clean the room by wiping down the surfaces with a damp cloth rather than a duster.

It is unlikely that you will be keen to apply these principles in the rest of the house unless your child has severe eczema or asthma as well. Bear them in mind, none the less. Choose linoleum or similar flooring whenever possible, and cut down the use of woolly rugs, velvet curtains and so on. Vacuum as often as possible, but remember that dust mite droppings do not become airborne unless disturbed. Cleaning procedures are likely to put up thousands of these particles, and they take a little time to settle. For this reason, you should keep your child well away when you are cleaning, and if dust has been disturbed keep your child out of that particular room for a few hours. Vacuum cleaners are preferable to a broom or brush and pan, but try to empty the bag more regularly than you normally would. Wipe down skirting boards, mantelpieces and sills frequently with a damp cloth.

In many children, eczema that is worst on the knees and at

the top of the backs of the thighs seems to have a special association with allergy to the house dust mite. I suspect that this is because sitting on settees and kneeling on carpets results in the particularly harmful combination of contact with house dust mite droppings and friction. If your child does sit on upholstered chairs or play on carpeted floors, have an old sheet that can be placed under them and be regularly washed.

Although dry air is disliked by the house dust mite, you would have to keep the central heating on for 24 hours a day throughout the year to have a really significant effect on them. Nevertheless, rising damp and other sources of unwanted moisture should be dealt with. Ducted air heating tends to make matters worse by constantly disturbing the air and raising the dust particles.

Interest has recently been renewed in the possibility of eradicating house dust mites by using chemicals. Those which simply kill the mites are generally too toxic for home use. There will, however, soon be available an agent which reduces the house dust mite population in a much more subtle way. This agent is known as Tymasil. It contains an antifungal compound called natamycin. Now, although I said earlier that house dust mites eat shed particles of human skin, the situation is now known to be slightly more complicated than this. What actually happens, as far as we can see, is that a mould-like fungus known as Aspergillus forms on organic household debris such as skin scales, and it is in fact this fungus which is eaten by the house dust mite. The natamycin kills the fungus and denies the mite its staple diet. Tymasil will be available as a treatment for mattresses, but how effective it will actually prove in practice remains to be seen.

Although desensitising injections may occasionally be helpful for eczema caused by grass pollen, the same has not so far been shown to be true for house dust mite allergy. Nevertheless, it is certainly possible that such treatment would help some children, and this is an area in which research is needed.

Domestic Animals Cats are a very common cause of allergic

symptoms, and they frequently play an important part in eczema. The problem is not, as is widely believed, the cat's hair, but rather the small scales, known as 'dander', which are continually shed from the cat's skin. The length of the cat's coat is therefore immaterial, because the amount of dander shed is much the same in both long and short-haired varieties. Dried cat's saliva and urine are also highly allergenic, but tend to be less important because they are generally present in only small quantities. As in the case of pollens and house dust mites, both direct skin contact and inhalation may aggravate eczema. I suspect that skin contact is particularly important in the case of cat allergy, and one can often get clues that a child may be allergic to cats from the pattern of their eczema. Marked involvement of the backs of the thighs and the fronts of the knees is a suspicious feature in a household where there is a cat for exactly the same reasons I indicated in the case of house dust mite allergy. Children who stroke and cuddle cats may have eczema which is worst on the cheeks and hands.

In general, it is unwise to have a cat if one's child has eczema. Even if your child is not at first allergic to the cat, it is more than likely that sooner or later he will become so, and this may take the form of asthma as well as eczema. Some children become so highly allergic to cats that they can become ill if they so much as enter a room in which there has been a cat within the previous day or two. This is the kind of problem any parent would wish to avoid. If your child has eczema, it would therefore be wise to do without a cat. Although I love cats, if you already have one, I would advise you to get rid of it and look out for a friend or relative who is prepared to look after it to save you having to put it down. After the cat has left, any improvement in your child's eczema may only be gradual because it takes several weeks or even months to eliminate every last trace of the dander.

Curiously, dogs do not seem to be such a potent cause of allergy as cats. Nevertheless, they do often cause problems and, just like cats, they have no place in any household in which there is a child with eczema. Again, the main allergen is the dander, and whether the dog has long, short or curly hair is immaterial; nor does it make any difference if it is one of those breeds that don't shed hair at all. Saliva and urine are also allergenic, and some children will demonstrate their sensitivity very clearly by developing weals where they are licked.

In the past, horses were probably the most important animals of all in terms of allergies, not only because there were so many of them around but also because horse hair was widely used in fillings for furniture and bedding, and was even used in making the plaster on walls. If your child has much contact with horses, development of allergy is a definite risk and ideally such contact should be minimised in children with eczema.

Allergies to virtually all domesic mammals have been recorded, both to pet species such as rabbits, mice and guinea-pigs, and to farm animals such as sheep, pigs and cattle. Children with eczema should have as little as possible to do with all such animals, and if your child is desperate to have a pet, go for something like tropical fish in preference.

Allergy to birds may be a similar problem. Again it is dander and droppings that seem to be responsible rather than the feathers themselves. Children who appear to be allergic to feathers are usually reacting to the dander and the mites that are associated with them. That is why washable artificial fillings are preferable to feathers for pillows, duvets and cushions, at least in your child's own room. At one time it was thought that wool allergy was common in children with eczema. However, it has now become clear that the trouble with wool is rarely allergy as such, but a direct irritation of the skin by the fibres, a subject we will come back to later (see p. 110).

Moulds and Algae. Moulds are fungi and live by extracting nourishment from decomposing organic matter of all sorts; they generally thrive in damp conditions. It is their spores which are most likely to provoke allergic symptoms. These are the equivalent of seeds in the case of plants but are microscopic, several times smaller even than pollen grains but similarly dispersed in the air. Like house dust mites, moulds are present throughout the year, but are particularly numerous in the autumn. In the home, they flourish in damp cellars and wherever there is rising damp. Dry rot is a mould that occasionally causes allergy. Stored grain, fruit and vegetables tend to be heavily colonised by moulds. Moulds are also present in house dust. Outside, they particularly like rotting plant matter such as compost heaps or windfallen fruit, and animal manure. Most plants support quite a large population of moulds even when healthy; the bloom visible on many fruits is a fine layer of mould. Much of the allergy problems attributed to grass may be due to moulds living on its surface.

In fact, very little is known about the importance of mould allergy in eczema, but the possibility that it may contribute to your child's problems should be considered. Some precautions make sense. Eliminating damp from the house helps to reduce both the amount of mould and the number of house dust mites. Avoid storing large quantities of foods such as grain, beans, dried fruit and apples. Out of doors, avoid assembling large heaps of compost, and keep those you do have covered with polythene. Collect up windfallen fruit and dispose of it.

Algae are similar to moulds but are actually microscopic plants which live by photosynthesis. Like moulds, they are widespread outside but, in contrast, will be very little problem inside. Like moulds, they often grow on the surface of plants, and lichen is in fact a combination of moulds and algae growing together. Algal spores are similarly dispersed in the air, but when they do contribute to eczema it is probably more often the result of direct contact than inhalation. There is little that can be done to reduce the population of algae, but bear in mind that they may cause problems. I know a child whose eczema appears to be aggravated by climbing trees, and it is likely that lichens on the bark are responsible. Children who itch after contact with grass may be reacting to algae (or moulds) rather than to pollen, and you should suspect that this is the case if grass seems to be troublesome outside the pollen season.

Anti-allergy Drugs

In Chapter 2, we considered the reaction that occurs when an antigen encounters its specific IgE antibodies on the surface of a mast cell. The cell is triggered to discharge substances that cause inflammation, including histamine (p. 11). Almost all children with eczema are atopic, i.e. they produce excessive amounts of IgE antibodies in response to common antigens. Many children who do not have eczema are also atopic; some will have asthma, some will have hayfever, but some will be entirely well. All these atopic children have mast cells that are highly sensitive and liable to discharge their contents readily on exposure to the appropriate antigen. This sensitive (i.e. allergic) state is detectable by skin testing (p. 8). Mast cell sensitivity in the lungs appears to be important in causing asthma, and mast cell sensitivity in the nose and eyes appears to be responsible for hayfever. Mast cell sensitivity is the cause of the skin wealing some people experience after eating particular foods, but its role in eczema is unclear, since the result of mast cell discharge in the skin is wealing and not eczema. Nevertheless, some drugs have been developed in the last few years which seem, in the laboratory at least, capable of preventing mast cells discharging their contents so readily when antigen meets antibody on their surface. For this reason, these drugs are often referred to as mast cell 'stabilisers'. The best known, and to date the most effective of these, is known as sodium cromoglycate. This drug has proved helpful in many cases of asthma, for which it is given by inhalation in a form called Intal. Other preparations of sodium cromoglycate called Rynacrom and Opticrom are often useful when given respectively in the nose and eye for hayfever. Sodium cromoglycate has also been tried in eczema by applying it to the skin in the form of an ointment. After initially encouraging reports, it now seems that it is ineffective when used in this way. It may simply be that insufficient amounts of the drug succeed in getting through to the mast cells because of the skin's barrier effect. Alternatively, it may be that sufficient does get through, but then fails to help simply because mast cells are not responsible for eczema.

If sodium cromoglycate is given by mouth, very little enters the blood, almost certainly insufficient to have any effect on distant organs like the skin. Given this way, however, it may be able to exert a local effect on the lining of the intestines. I mentioned in Chapter 5 (p. 27) that children with eczema have intestines which appear to allow in more intact food antigens than those of normal children. It seems that a damaging reaction in the intestines themselves may be at least partly responsible for this increased permeability. This allergic reaction would almost certainly involve IgE antibody and mast cells. If this initial reaction in the intestines could be prevented, one might be able to prevent the eczema which appears to be its consequence. Again, some early studies suggested that oral sodium cromoglycate (marketed as Nalcrom) might be helpful in atopic eczema. Unfortunately it now seems that this early optimism was unjustified; Nalcrom seems to have little beneficial effect in children with eczema, but why this should be the case is uncertain. This is a familiar problem in medicine: a drug does not work when theoretically it should. More research is needed to discover why this is. It may be, for example, that the drug does reduce the absorption of intact proteins to, say, one half of what it would otherwise be, but that this is simply not enough to make any noticeable difference.

More recently, several new drugs of this type have been developed and these await careful appraisal in eczema. Most of them differ from sodium cromoglycate in being absorbed in reasonable amounts into the bloodstream. Whether this will make them more effective or only more toxic remains to be seen. Even so, there is room for guarded optimism that some of these drugs will prove helpful.

Avoiding Irritants

We considered the harmful effects of cutaneous irritants in Chapter 5 (see p. 32). The mechanisms by which such irritants contribute to eczema have nothing in common with allergic reactions, and although irritants undoubtedly play an important role in atopic eczema they are not capable of causing it on their own. Allergy is the 'sine qua non' of atopic eczema, though the responsible allergens will differ from child to child. The irritants which further aggravate the situation are, on the other hand, always much the same. Careful observation will often give strong clues to those that are causing problems to your own child. Some are easily avoided, others only with difficulty. I will tackle them by suggesting some general rules, but how assiduously you should follow these rules must depend on the severity of your child's eczema.

(a) Avoid *soap and detergents* when washing your child, similarly soapy additives such as *foaming agents* or *bubble baths*. If you ever *have* to use soap, use a baby soap or a non-alkaline soap such as Neutrogena.

(b) Do not let your child play with *water* for long periods. Before playing with water or *swimming*, it is a good idea to cover the skin with grease to protect it; white soft paraffin (Vaseline) is ideal for this purpose. Immediately afterwards, a shower or bath with emulsifying ointment (p. 44) is also helpful.

(c) Don't let your child handle *irritant foods* if his hands are affected – particularly oranges, lemons, grapefruits and onions. Peel oranges yourself. Tomatoes, apples and pears are less irritating, but these should likewise be handled as little as possible. If your child gets food all over his face when eating, avoid giving him these irritant fruits and vegetables; the same applies to spicy foods such as tomato ketchup.

(d) When dressing your child, avoid having *pure wool or nylon* next to the skin. Wherever possible, any clothing that comes into direct contact with the skin should be pure cotton or a high cotton mixture. A good range of 100% cotton clothes is obtainable by mail order from Cotton On, 29, North Clifton Street, Lytham FY8 5HW, Tel: 0253–736611. Socks containing a high ratio of cotton are made by Clarks, and can be bought in shops selling their shoes. Remember that wrists and necks are likely to come into contact with pullovers, whatever is worn underneath, and these areas often suffer greatly as a result. For the same reasons, try not to let your child's skin come into direct contact with carpets, particularly synthetic ones. As I suggested earlier in connection with house dust mite allergy, a cotton sheet should be placed over the carpet where your child is playing.

(e) Do not overheat your child. Remember that *heat* is one of the greatest enemies of anyone with eczema.

Let us look at this problem more closely. Human beings need to maintain a constant body temperature. Heat loss through the skin must therefore be precisely matched by heat production. Heat is produced mainly by the liver, but also as a byproduct of muscle activity. This system has both a coarse and a fine control. Coarse control is the function of thyroid hormones. If the body's temperature is too low, thyroid hormone production is stepped up and the liver responds by increasing its heat output. Nevertheless, a fine control is needed in addition, because there would be a considerable lag between any change in body temperature and the resulting change in liver heat output if one had to depend entirely on the thyroid gland. This fine control must provide for a more rapid response. A sudden fall in body temperature may be compensated for by shivering, an involuntary mechanism that takes advantage of the heat produced by muscle activity. If the body's temperature rises, heat loss can be increased further still by sweating; the evaporation of sweat produces quick cooling. Heat loss by both these mechanisms is reduced by clothing and by high air temperatures.

This whole system bears a close resemblance to a domestic central heating system. The boiler is the liver, the circulating water is the blood and the pipework is the blood vessels. Coarse control is achieved by turning the boiler up or down. When it comes to fine control, the equivalent of shivering is turning on an electric fire. The windows are like the skin; open them and heat loss is accelerated; close them and it is reduced.

In most people, this system is fairly finely balanced. But in children with eczema, which affects large areas of skin, it can become disturbed. The problem is caused by the huge heat losses that occur through these areas of inflamed skin. Because of this inflammation, large volumes of blood are flowing very close to the surface; this is why they look red. To compensate for such high losses, the liver produces more heat. This is much the same as having all the windows in your house open on a winter's day; you would need to turn the boiler right up to keep the house warm. This of course requires extra fuel, which is why children with severe eczema tend to have good appetites. They are making heat very much faster than other children, and as long as they are also losing it faster, their condition remains stable. But if the heat loss is in any way prevented, the child will quickly overheat. This may happen if the air temperature is high, if they are wearing too many clothes, if a bath is too hot, or if they exert themselves physically. It may even happen if they have a hot meal. This is exactly what would occur if the boiler had been turned up to compensate for the windows being open, and you suddenly shut all the windows. This unsatisfactory and unstable situation is aggravated by the fact that sweating tends to be impaired in eczematous skin, so that this emergency system for cooling the body is less effective. The inflammation appears to damage the ducts that lead up to the surface from the sweat glands. As well as causing blockage of these ducts, the eczematous process seems to make these ducts leaky, as a result of which some sweat seeps out into the already inflammed tissues. This seepage of sweat causes further irritation. As a result, when the child overheats the skin may become unbearably itchy.

I hope that all this helps to explain some of the problems of heat regulation in children with eczema. Your child needs to be able to lose the extra heat that is being produced. To help prevent overheating, rooms should be kept cool, below 20°C (68°F). Bedrooms particularly should be kept cool. Baths should be cooler than you would like yourself. Be very careful not to overdress your child; he would rather be slightly too cold than too hot.

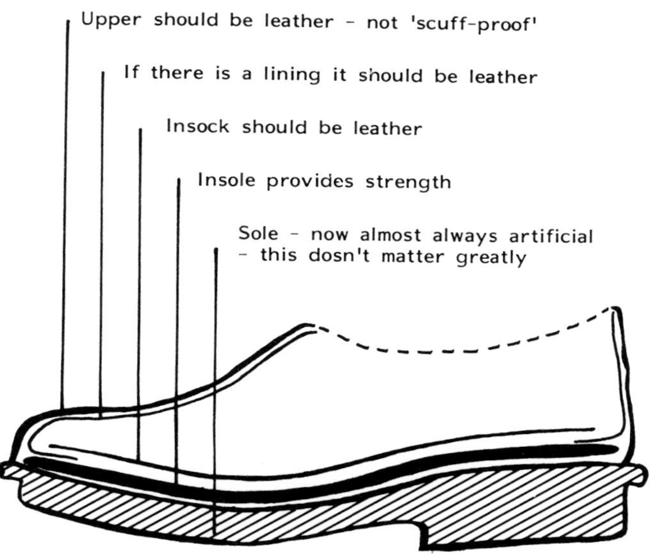

Fig 7.27a Diagram of shoe cut through lengthways, to show the various parts used and of what they should ideally be made if your child has eczema of the feet.

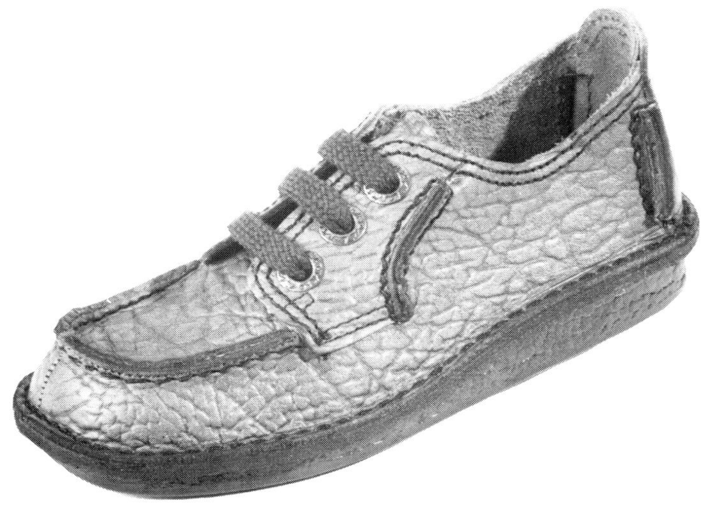

Fig. 7.27b An example of an ideal shoe for the child with eczema of the feet. 'Oberon' by Clarks Ltd.

(f) Pay careful attention to *footwear* if your child has a problem with eczema of the feet (Fig 7.27a, b).

Hot sweaty conditions make foot eczema worse and may be the reason the feet were affected in the first place. Footwear should be dry and permeable to air. The foot's worst enemy in this respect is the 'trainer' shoe, which is usually made of plastic and completely airtight. If your child has eczema of the feet, you should outlaw this type of shoe. Unfortunately, the right type of shoe is expensive. It should have leather uppers. If there is a lining, this should also be leather and should be glued by the spot method, not be a continuous layer of adhesive. The in-sock should also be made of leather. It may be difficult to check all these things without actually taking the shoe apart – not generally a popular move in shoe shops! The safest thing is to buy shoes made by a manufacturer that takes trouble to get these things right. Clarks are one of the leaders in this respect, though not all their shoes have leather in-socks. Nevertheless, I understand that they have arranged to make these available to their agents, who will fit them on request at no extra cost. Clarks' 'Movers' range are particularly suitable as they are highly permeable, being made of pigskin without any lining and with a leather in-sock. Good leather sandals are best of all, though clearly they will not be appropriate throughout the year.

Avoid any shoe, even if it has leather uppers, if it has been treated with a scuff-proof finish because this reduces permeability. If your child's shoes do not have leather in-socks, you can help to increase air circulation in the shoe by buying an untreated leather in-sock to insert over the existing in-sock. These may be difficult to find, and a cork in-sock is the next best thing so long as it does not make the shoe too tight. Many shops also sell special 'ventilators' which do the same job.

If the same shoes are worn day after day, there will be a gradual steady build-up of moisture in the leather. This should be avoided by giving shoes a day's rest for every day they are worn. This also makes for additional expense, but does have the advantage of extending the life of the shoes.

Socks act as a wick, drawing moisture up from the foot to the ankle and lower leg from where it evaporates away. Long socks do this better than short ones, and those made of natural fibres do it better than artificial ones.

One word of caution on the subject of foot eczema. A very small number of children are actually allergic to shoe constituents, most commonly chromate which is used in leather tanning, or the rubber chemicals used in shoe adhesives. This is the type of allergy which can be investigated by special skin tests called patch tests (see p. 6). This kind of allergy is rare in children, but you should be suspicious if your child's eczema affects the feet predominantly.

(g) Avoid the use of plastic pants for babies, because these encourage hot humid conditions in the nappy area. Apart from the irritant effect, such conditions provide a strong stimulus to the multiplication of micro-organisms which can make eczema in this area worse.

In many infants, eczema starts in the nappy area. Most babies with such eczema (doctors usually call this 'napkin dermatitis') will never get atopic eczema; in these cases the rash seems to be an irritant reaction to urine and faeces often compounded by the effects of plastic pants, without the underlying allergies of the child with atopic eczema. In a smaller number of cases, what seems to start as ordinary napkin dermatitis gradually spreads and subsequently appears on the face and body. In some of these children, this more general eruption will clear up as soon as the rash in the nappy area gets better. In others, the rash will gradually take on the typical features of atopic eczema, and will remain elsewhere even after it has cleared from the nappy area itself. Exactly what is going on in such cases is not fully understood. Personally, I think that some of those children who are going to develop atopic eczema in any case will first get it in the nappy area, simply because it is localised to this site by an irritant effect. Other children get napkin dermatitis pure and simple, and are in no special danger of developing full-blown atopic eczema. Unfortunately, the two conditions are impossible to distinguish at first.

If your baby has eczema in the nappy area, certain measures are likely to help. Never let a wet or soiled nappy remain unchanged any longer than is absolutely necessary. Only use plastic pants or disposable nappies when it is essential to do so – for example, when going out. Avoid paper liners; use muslin ones if possible. Leave nappies off completely whenever practicable. Do not use 'biological' washing powders, and rinse thoroughly; machine-washing is ideal because most machines rinse well. Do not use fabric conditioners because these leave residual chemicals in the nappy. Tumble-drying is best because it leaves the nappies softer and more absorbent.

(h) If possible, use soft water to wash or bath your child. Eczema is commoner in those parts of the country where the water is hard, and many parents have told me that buying a domestic water softener has had a beneficial and occasionally dramatic effect on their child's skin. Exactly why hardness in water should be an irritant is unclear. To soften your child's bath water does not mean that you have to invest in a complete domestic water softening system costing hundreds of pounds. You can buy a portable softener such as the one illustrated in Fig 7.28. (Further information is available from

Fig. 7.28 Portable water softener, by Permutit.

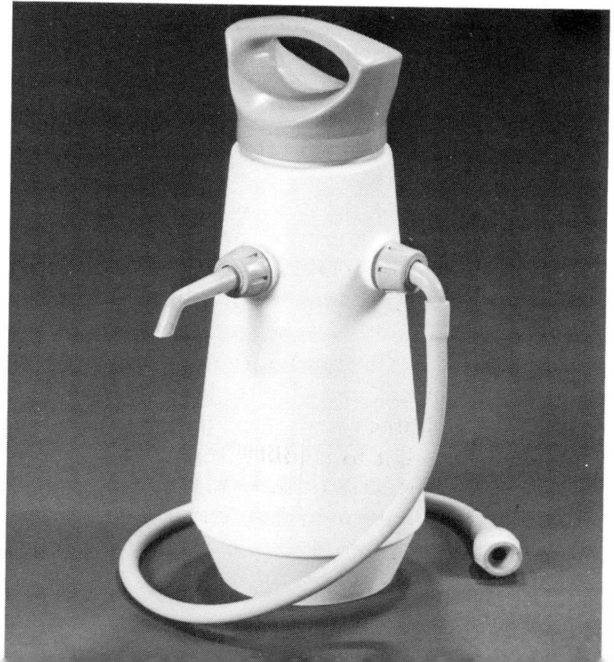

the makers, Houseman Ltd., Permutit Domestic Division, The Priory, Burnham, Slough SL1 7LS, who are prepared to offer a 25% discount to eczema patients if they can provide a letter from their doctor.)

(i) Cut your child's fingernails regularly. Scratching is, in a sense, the most ferocious irritant of all; keeping the nails short helps to reduce the damage. Wearing mitts at night provides further protection. The problem of scratching, and parents' attitude to it is discussed in Chapter 10.

(j) Protect your child's skin from extremes of climate.

Cold is a powerful irritant to skin. Cover up as much of your child's skin as possible before going outside in cold weather, particularly when it is windy. Gloves are especially important. Put a good layer of a moisturiser such as white soft paraffin (Vaseline) or emulsifying ointment on exposed skin as this will provide some protection. As we have already considered, high temperatures are also very irritating; therefore dress your child lightly in hot weather and discourage too much rushing around when it is hot. Occasionally direct sunlight helps eczema, but more often it proves irritating.

(k) Consider the use of humidifiers.

The air inside our houses tends to be dry in the winter, especially when it is cold. Central heating greatly exacerbates the situation. While dry air has a bad effect on the skin in general, on eczematous skin it can be very detrimental. Obviously you don't want conditions to be frankly damp, but gentle humidification can help a lot. Humidity can be increased in several ways – by having plants, by burning paraffin stoves, by leaving bowls of water around – but the best way is to use either electric humidifiers or the type that are hung on radiators. If you want to take this seriously, buy a hygrometer, which is an instrument that measures humidity; hair hygrometers are probably the most suitable type for home use. Try to keep the reading above 55%.

Other Approaches to Treatment

Homeopathy

Homeopathy is an approach to medicine that was developed in Europe about 100 years ago. There are two principal features which distinguish it from mainstream medicine. The first is the concept of treating like with like. Thus jaundice, in which the patient goes yellow, is treated with gold, and eczema, an eruption of the skin, is treated with sulphur, a product of volcanic eruptions. The second feature of homeopathy is that the remedies are given in minute quantities. The idea is to give an infinitely small dose. These infinitesimal doses do, of course, have the great virtue of being harmless, and the reason that homeopathic medicine first caught on in the nineteenth century has, I suspect, quite a lot to do with this freedom from hazard. At a time when doctors could do little for their patients, and when their treatments could prove even more unpleasant than the diseases they were used to treat, the gentle approach of the homeopathist would be safer and more attractive. I have great sympathy for this approach, but I must confess I find myself unable to grasp the rationale of homeopathy. My own feeling is that it is probably the least helpful of the 'alternative' approaches in the treatment of eczema.

Hypnosis

Hypnosis can be valuable in treating any disease whose effects can be modified by the mind. A good example is high blood pressure. It has been shown that most people can lower their own blood pressure by a conscious effort to relax mentally and physically, and a similar method can be used to treat duodenal ulcers by reducing the stomach's secretion of acid. The hypnotist can teach his patients to gain a degree of mental control over body functions. In eczema, the symptom of itching is highly susceptible to psychological influences. The hypnotist aims at giving the eczema sufferer the ability to control itching by willpower, and there are various ways in which this may be done. A popular one is to get the patient to 'channel' the irritation into one part of the body, say the little finger. Then, by squeezing this finger the symptom is controlled. There is no doubt that this approach can be useful. It is very satisfying for the eczema sufferer to feel that real control of his disease can be achieved. It is a treatment without side effects, but clearly it will not suit everyone. In particular, it will not be appropriate for the very young, and I imagine there can be few children under five years of age who would benefit from it.

Acupuncture

Acupuncture is an integral part of an entirely distinct Chinese system of medicine, built up over many hundreds of years. The way it works is unknown, though it has been suggested that it modifies the patient's perception of unpleasant sensation by altering the levels of certain natural body chemicals known as 'endorphins'. These are chemicals which have effects similar to morphine, the most potent of all known pain-relieving drugs. The traditional Chinese belief is that all illness reflects a disturbance of the natural harmony of the body, and that acupuncture helps to correct this.

Most people think of acupuncture as meaning needles, but there are other ways of producing a similar effect. Finger pressure is used in the technique of acupressure. There is even a technique of laser acupuncture. Another alternative method is to apply heat locally by burning a kind of herbal cigarette close to the skin. The value of any of these forms of acupuncture in eczema remains unestablished, but it seems to me that there is no reason why it should not be helpful in some cases.

Evening Primrose Oil

Over 40 years ago it was first suggested that children with eczema might be deficient in what are known as 'essential fatty acids'. Fatty acids are the building bricks with which fats are made by the body, and they are therefore somewhat analogous to the amino-acids of which proteins are made (see p. 26). Some fatty acids can be made by the body itself; others cannot, and these must be absorbed into the body direct from the diet – these are the 'essential' fatty acids. Fats are usually thought of in the context of obesity, but as well as being deposited as an energy source for use in emergencies fats play a vital role in the body's everyday functions. They are one of the most important constituents of the membranes that envelop every living cell, and they are a component of the waxy surface layer of normal skin. If one is deprived of essential fatty acids, this surface layer cracks up like sun-dried mud on a parched lake bed, and the skin becomes scaly and irritable. This is not quite the same thing as eczema, and it seems improbable that eczema could be caused by nothing more than a deficiency of these essential fatty acids. Nevertheless, over the years there have been sporadic reports of successful treatment of atopic eczema by oils rich in essential fatty acids. The oil extracted from the seeds of the evening primrose (*Oenethera biennis*) is a particularly good source of essential fatty acids, and some recent research has indicated that it may be beneficial in atopic eczema. Though the effect appears likely to be a relatively small one, it would nevertheless be of considerable interest because it could give some additional clues about the cause of the disease.

The question of whether this oil is really helpful in atopic eczema is at present unanswered, but it is clear that it is no miracle cure. It is certainly harmless and can be bought in many health food shops under the brand name Efamol. The ideal dose is probably between four and eight 0.5g capsules daily, depending on the size of the child. Studies so far suggest that evening primrose oil is more likely to be helpful in adults with atopic eczema than in children. My own limited experience has not been promising, but in individual cases this treatment appears to be worth a try.

Hospital Admission: Why Does it Work?

When eczema gets out of control the question arises whether the child should be admitted to hospital. In the short term, hospital admission may be beneficial both to the affected child and to the family, but it represents no kind of long-term solution. When weighing up the pros and cons of admitting a child with eczema, most dermatologists and paediatricians will consider the interests of the rest of the family as much as those of the child himself. Living with a severely eczematous child who is getting steadily worse in spite of all efforts can be an extremely harassing experience for parents, as many readers will know. Faced with the unrelieved suffering of their child, the hopelessness felt by parents is frequently heightened by lack of sleep and by disagreements about treatment. Brothers and sisters feel neglected, and may be disturbed by their parents' obvious distress. This distress in its turn becomes a major factor in further aggravating the eczema of the affected child, and the family can become caught up in a vicious spiral. It is in these conditions that admission can be most effective. The child with eczema is taken out of what has become a stressful home into the relatively relaxed atmosphere of hospital where he is no longer the centre of attention and anxiety. The family can rest and recover their sapped strength.

Parents are often amazed at how effective hospital admission can be in clearing up a bad attack of eczema. Indeed, it can be aggravating to see the treatments that failed at home now appearing to work so well. The reason for the improvement in the eczema probably owes less to the treatment itself than everybody thinks, including the doctors and nurses. As I have already suggested, the most important influence is often the change of scene itself, and the child's removal from what has – through nobody's fault – become an electrified home environment. Though you may think this sounds harsh and old-fashioned, I believe that the benefits of admission can be lessened by excessive visiting by parents. I see it as an opportunity for everyone to get a break from one another and rebuild their reserves. Visiting is obviously important, but each visit should be short, no more than an hour or so. This is a generalisation, of course, and there will inevitably be times when a child with eczema is admitted and the parents' presence is important.

There may be other reasons why a spell in hospital can help a child with eczema. Levels of house dust are generally low, for example, and there are no furry animals. Although a short stay in hospital can for all these reasons be a good idea as a temporary measure, it can never become a substitute for good home treatment. One hears of children who spend more time in than out of hospital; this is a bad thing.

8 Complications of Atopic Eczema

Eczema Herpeticum

In Chapters 4 and 6 we considered the colonisation and infection of eczematous skin by bacteria. Certain viruses may also secure a foothold in skin affected by eczema, where they may provoke dramatic and occasionally dangerous infections. The virus most likely to do this is known as *Herpesvirus hominis* or the herpes simplex virus. This virus causes the common cold sore that many people get around the lips, though few of them realise that a virus is responsible. Just as in the case of measles or chickenpox, it is unusual for anyone to escape infection with *Herpesvirus hominis*, though once one has had it an immunity is developed which provides protection from further attacks. The initial infection with *Herpesvirus hominis* is most commonly in the mouth and on the lips, where it causes crops of small blisters and ulcers which may be very painful. Most of these initial infections are never identified; many are mild and go unnoticed; others are simply not recognised for what they are. The body's defence mechanisms get on top of the infection and mop up all the virus, or almost all. Virus reaching the body from the outside is quickly dealt with thereafter and will fail to become established. Nevertheless, small numbers of viruses often linger on in guerrilla-like fashion, hidden away from the body's defences in the nerves that provide sensation around the lips. Most of the time the defence system keeps them locked away in these sites, unable to venture forth. However, when the body is run down by other illness for example, these viruses take the opportunity to travel down the nerves into the skin around the lips where they set up a localised infection. When the body defences realise what is happening the infection is quickly dealt with. Unfortunately, small numbers of viruses may hold out for years in their outposts in these nerves, so that infections of this type may be a recurrent problem. They are known as herpes labialis, or cold sores. Sometimes, just a cold wind or even strong sunlight on the lips can be enough to reactivate the infection.

The problem with cold sores is that they provide a source of viruses that can start off infections in children who have never encountered them previously, and who have therefore no protection. Although the initial infection with *Herpesvirus hominis* is normally in the mouth, in children with certain skin diseases, and especially eczema, it may take place instead on affected areas of skin. If the eczema is severe and extensive the infection can spread rapidly, and the situation can become a serious one. Infection of eczematous skin with *Herpesvirus hominis* is known as eczema herpeticum.

If this happens to your child, you may not immediately realise the cause of the problem. The virus infection causes a rash which is superimposed upon the eczema itself. This rash consists of clusters of small blisters (known as vesicles), each blister usually not being more than 2mm or 3mm across (Fig 8.1). At first they are filled with clear fluid; later this often turns

Fig 8.1 Eczema herpeticum. Typical clusters of umbilicated blisters on the face at the earliest stage of the infection.

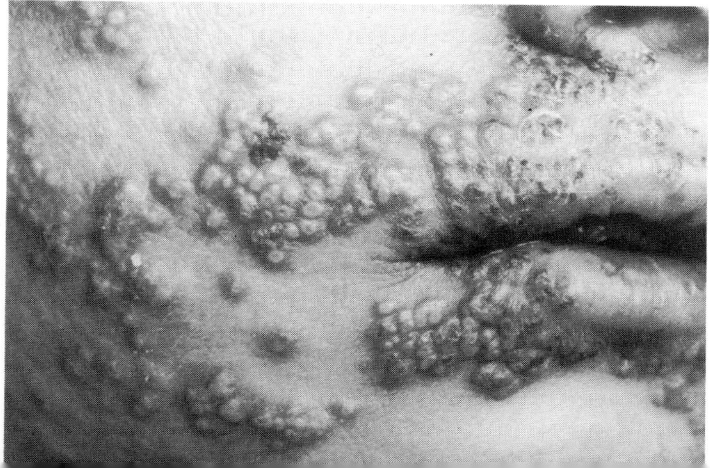

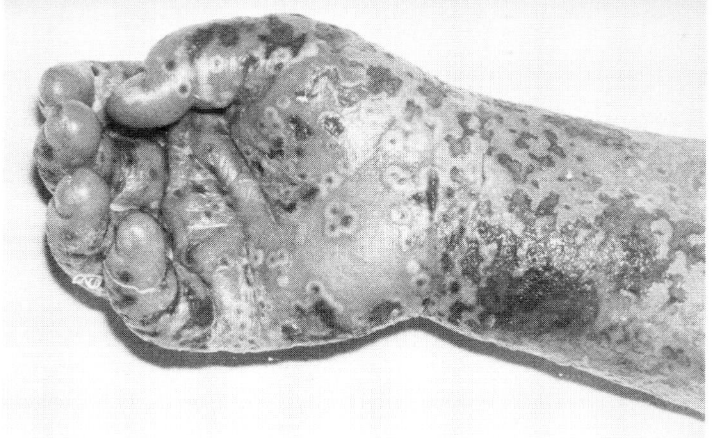

Fig. 8.2 Eczema herpeticum. Some of the original umbilicated blisters are still visible near the wrist. Elsewhere, the blisters have broken, leaving extensive raw areas. This is a particularly nasty example, most attacks are much less severe.

to pus. Many of the blisters develop a small central depression, and this is highly characteristic. The tops of these rather fragile blisters tend to be scratched away fairly quickly, leaving raw weeping or pus-filled areas, which later become encrusted over (Fig. 8.2). Viruses can easily enter the blood from infected areas of skin, and from there they can be transported to distant areas of skin and also to internal organs. This is what makes eczema herpeticum potentially dangerous and, without wishing to cause alarm, I feel that readers should know that the condition is occasionally lethal. Fortunately, this is extremely rare. Recently a drug has become available, known as acyclovir, which can control the multiplication of this virus. For the present, the drug has to be given intravenously and can therefore be administered only in hospitals, where its use is reserved for those children who are considered to be severely affected.

Clearly, you should try to keep any child with eczema away from anyone who has a cold sore. If a member of your family ever does have one, it should be kept covered and that person should avoid physical contact with the eczematous child until the cold sore has gone. If your child's eczema ever gets worse rapidly for no apparent reason, the reason may be eczema herpeticum. Suspect it particularly if there is an obvious change in the quality of the eczema, and especially if you see the clusters of small blisters I described above. Seek medical advice quickly if your child is obviously unwell or has a high temperature.

Because eczema herpeticum is a reaction to the child's first encounter with the virus, immunity will follow; second attacks are rare and when they do occur are usually mild. The child may subsequently suffer from cold sores but, because immunity will have been developed, there is little danger of it spreading more widely on the skin.

A similar infection in eczematous skin may occur with the virus used for smallpox vaccination (see p. 136), but fortunately it very rarely happens with any other virus.

Allergic Rhinitis

'Rhinitis' is the medical term for inflammation of the membrane lining the inside of the nose. Rhinitis is remarkably common in children with eczema, in whom it may cause a variety of symptoms including a 'runny' nose, sneezing, difficulty in breathing through the nose, and snoring. These all result from inflammation of the nasal lining (the nasal 'mucosa'), which becomes swollen and irritable. Allergic rhinitis is the term used when this inflammation is caused by an allergic reaction; usually the allergy is to airborne particles which are breathed in and land on the nasal mucosa. If pollen alone is responsible, symptoms will occur only during the pollen season, causing what is popularly known as 'hayfever', or seasonal allergic rhinitis. If house dust mites, mould spores or animal dander are responsible, symptoms will tend to occur more or less the whole year round; this condition is known as perennial allergic rhinitis.

There is very strong evidence that mast cells (p. 11) play a leading part in allergic rhinitis. When a pollen grain lands on the nasal mucosa, the wet surface causes the antigenic proteins within the pollen grain to dissolve. These proteins can then be absorbed through the mucosa, where they come into contact with the mast cells. If the child is allergic to pollen, they will make IgE antibodies against pollen proteins and these will have become attached to the mast cells. Contact between the proteins and mast cells primed in this way leads to the release from the mast cells of substances causing inflammation, such as histamine. In fact, antigenic proteins which reach these mast cells via the bloodstream – food proteins, for example – can probably also cause this condition. In young children it is possible that food allergy may be quite a common cause of rhinitis, though airborne antigens are likely to be more important.

Inflammation of the nasal mucosa causes it to exude fluid, which causes a runny nose. Just as in eczematous skin, the blood flow is increased and this may cause nose bleeds. Swelling of the mucosa often causes blockage of air flow through the passages of the nose. Affected children may be able to breathe only through the mouth and this can in turn lead to other problems such as sore throats in the mornings. Nasal obstruction may also cause snoring. The lining of the nose extends into air spaces in the bones of the face, known as 'sinuses'. Swelling of the lining of these sinuses can cause pain in the face or headaches. Still more problems may be caused by blockage of the so-called Eustachian tube. This is a channel connecting the air space inside each eardrum with the nose. Its function is simply to equalise pressure between the two sides of the eardrum. The clicking sensation in the ears when one comes down a mountain or descends a tall building in a lift is caused by a succession of closings and openings of this tube. Its own lining is continuous with that of the nose and, if this lining is swollen, the channel may become blocked. This may cause ear problems, including infections causing earache ('otitis media') and hearing problems, both of which will need treatment in their own right.

Treatment is unnecessary for minor degrees of rhinitis, but if breathing through either nostril becomes completely blocked or if your child develops earache or any difficulty with hearing, you should consult your doctor. In the short term, the nasal blockage can be relieved by nose drops or sprays containing drugs that reduce blood flow, and thus reduce the swelling. These include such preparations as Otrivine and Iliadin. Although effective when used for short periods, these drugs may aggravate the condition if used continuously. Fairly effective long-term treatment may be obtained by using the mast cell stabilising drug, sodium cromoglycate (see p. 108) (Lomusol, Rynacrom) though regular treatment, six times daily, is essential. If symptoms are very severe, a corticosteroid preparation is justified and there are several of these now available, of which Beconase is a good example. Your doctor will be able to assess the necessity for any treatment and weigh up the pros and cons of the various approaches.

Allergic Conjunctivitis

The conjunctiva is a thin, almost invisible, membrane covering the eye. Inflammation of this membrane is called conjunctivitis and allergy is commonly responsible. Allergic conjunctivitis is, like allergic rhinitis, common in children with eczema, and similarly may be either seasonal, usually due to pollen allergy, or perennial, due to other allergies. The seasonal variety is a characteristic component of hayfever; this is the more usual form in children with eczema. Conjunctivitis causes redness, watering of the eyes and a rather gritty sensation. Like rhinitis, it can be treated with drugs causing decreased blood flow such as Otrivine-Antistin, by sodium cromoglycate (Opticrom) or corticosteroids (for example, Hydrocortistab, Predsol).

Cataract and Keratoconus

Unlike allergic conjunctivitis these are rare ocular complications of atopic eczema. Cataracts are opacities which may appear for a variety of reasons in the lens of the eye. Children with eczema may develop a rather characteristic type of cataract, though fortunately these rarely cause significant interference with vision. Since their cause is not established, little can be done to prevent the problems they occasionally cause. The best course of action is to have your child's vision tested every year. If they do interfere significantly with vision, the affected lens can be removed but I would emphasise how rarely such action is necessary.

Keratoconus is a weakness of the cornea, the clear window at the front of the eye. Why such a weakness should occur is unknown but it is relatively common in children with eczema. Occasionally it causes some deterioration in vision in children who have, or have had, eczema around puberty. This can usually be corrected by the use of glasses, but if very severe may require a corneal graft. Again, regular eye testing will alert one to the possibility of keratoconus.

Infraorbital Fold

Most children with eczema have an extra crease in the skin below their eyes, which has the effect of making them look tired; it tends to be associated with rather a bluish tint to the skin around the eyes, which heightens the effect. There are several theories on the cause of this extra crease. For example, it has been suggested that congestion of the nose and sinuses, due to allergic rhinitis, leads to a build-up of fluid (oedema) in the upper part of the face and that this is responsible. Against this idea is the fact that many eczematous children have this fold without any real sign of rhinitis. Possibly a better explanation is that it is in fact due to a mild degree of eczema which in itself causes swelling in the skin without any obvious involvement of the skin surface. A mild degree of lichenification (p. 21) due to rubbing would add to the swollen appearance.

Pallor

Most children with eczema have a curious pallid hue to their skin, and this is often mistaken for anaemia. This pallor appears to result from a somewhat reduced flow of blood through the skin in areas which are not affected by eczema. Where there is eczema, of course, the flow is increased. The significance of this altered pattern of blood flow is unknown, though some research workers believe that it may provide important clues about the basis of atopic eczema itself. It may, on the other hand, be due to the effects of chemicals released into the blood during the inflammatory process, and therefore may be an effect of the eczema rather than anything to do with its cause.

Nail Damage

Nail problems are a common complication of atopic eczema. Figure 8.3 is a diagram of what the end of a finger would look like, sliced through, and I hope it makes these problems easier

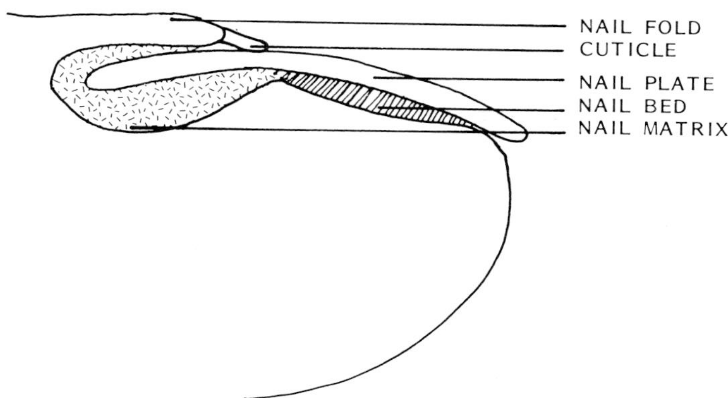

Fig. 8.3 Diagram of the end of a finger, cut through lengthways to show the nail.

to understand. The nail plate is made of exactly the same material as the surface layer of the rest of the skin – keratin – and the specialised part of the epidermis that produces it is known as the nail matrix. As it is formed, it is pushed outwards, stuck down on its underside by an adhesive tissue called the nail bed. The nail matrix is really an invagination of the skin, which forms a kind of pocket from which the nail emerges. The entrance to the pocket is sealed by the nail bed below and by the cuticle above. The cuticle is particularly prone to damage if the fingers are affected by eczema. When the bond between the cuticle and the nail plate is broken, the route is open for bacteria and yeasts to get into the pocket. This is just the sort of warm, moist place they like, and the resulting infection, known as paronychia, will damage the top of the nail, producing a series of transverse depressions and ridges in the nail. Where the infection is more intense, it may cause more severe damage to the surface of the nail.

Another type of problem can occur as a consequence of getting debris caught under the nail while scratching. If this debris contains bacteria and yeasts, infection can get a grip under the nail plate and this may be very painful. Such infections can cause the nail plate to lose its adherence to the nail bed, and occasionally nails are lost in this way. They will, however, always grow again. Avoiding this type of infection is another good reason for keeping the nails as short as possible to prevent anything becoming lodged underneath.

Lymph Nodes

In my introductory chapter on the normal skin I briefly described the function of lymph nodes. Let us now take a closer look at these. All the tissues of the body are supplied with blood via the arteries. Most of this blood is then taken back to the heart and lungs in veins. Blood itself consists of various types of living cells, namely red cells, which carry oxygen and give blood its colour, and several distinct forms of white cells (see Chapter 3, p. 10), all suspended in a clear fluid known as serum. As it passes through the tiny blood vessels in the tissues, some of this serum seeps out to provide the fluid that bathes all the living cells in the body. This clear tissue fluid is called lymph. It is continuously being freshly produced, and is constantly being collected and passed back into the blood through a network of special channels which are distinct from blood vessels, the lymph vessels. On its way, the lymph is passed through a series of filters, which are small bean-like structures known as lymph nodes. Lymph is passed through these lymph nodes into larger and larger vessels until it flows back into the blood via a vein deep in the chest.

The most important part of the lymph node's work is to filter out bacteria, yeasts and viruses from the lymph, as these could be very dangerous if they were to enter the bloodstream. Under normal circumstances one is unaware of the activity of these little organs. Even so, when they are having to work really hard they often become enlarged and tender. This is a common problem in the lymph nodes that drain lymph from

Fig. 8.4 A swollen lymph node under the arm of a boy with eczema. Though uncomfortable, these swellings need cause no anxiety.

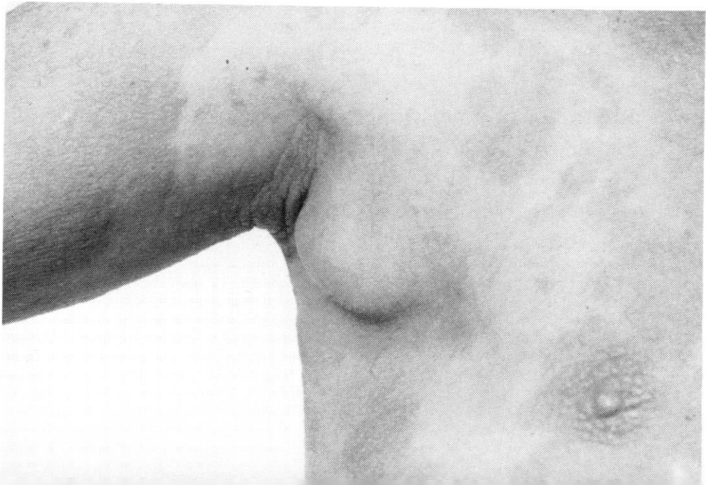

skin damaged by eczema. Parents are often worried by the painful lumps they notice in their children's groins, axillae (armpits) and necks (Fig. 8.4). These painful little lumps are, in a sense, a sign of health. They are a witness to a vigorous effort to protect your child from infection of the blood. Later on, when the skin improves, the lymph nodes will also settle down again.

Abdominal Pain

Children who have eczema seem to complain of tummy pains more often than other children, and the reason for this is unclear. There is certainly nothing to suggest that they have any serious cause. Just as eczema may be accompanied by painful allergic disorders of the nose and eye, it can probably be accompanied by painful allergic reactions in the gut. An alternative explanation is that these pains are caused by enlarged tender lymph nodes in the abdomen. On their way to the chest large numbers of lymph vessels pass through the abdomen, carrying lymph from the legs. Others carry lymph from the intestines themselves, and all this lymph passes through nodes in the abdomen. If these are inflamed they would cause deep-seated aching. They might be inflamed because they are filtering micro-organisms from the skin on the legs, or micro-organisms or foreign proteins that have got in through an unusually permeable intestine wall.

Whatever their cause, however, little can or need be done about such pains, but one must remember that children with eczema are just as liable to more serious diseases as other children. If the tummyache seems different, or worse than usual, a real problem such as appendicitis needs to be considered.

Urethritis

If the genital area is affected by eczema in children of either sex, the opening of the urinary canal, the urethra, may become inflamed. If this happens there may be a burning sensation when passing urine, and this can lead to the mistaken diagnosis of urinary infections such as cystitis (infection of the bladder). This problem is common and does not require treatment with antibiotics by mouth as urinary infections would. Application of corticosteroid cream around the urethral opening will often relieve the discomfort. Having said this, true urinary tract infections can of course occur in children with eczema, just as in other children, but they can be distinguished by examination of urine specimens by your doctor.

9 What About Immunisations?

The widespread confusion about immunisations in eczematous children is unjustified. Even doctors seem uncertain which immunisations should be given and which should not. The situation is not helped in the slightest by the vaccine manufacturers, whose literature seems to abound with vague warnings not to immunise children with unspecified 'allergies'. The truth is simple; eczematous children are not at special risk from immunisations, with the one important exception of smallpox vaccination.

It was well known to country folk over 200 years ago that anyone who had a disease called cow-pox appeared thereafter to be protected from smallpox, at that time a widespread and much-feared disease. Cow-pox, or 'vaccinia', is a viral disease which principally affects cattle, but humans can contract it as a result of handling an infected animal. In humans, the infection is generally mild, consisting of a single pustule which resolves spontaneously without any treatment. Edward Jenner (1749–1823) was the first person to give people cow-pox deliberately to protect them from smallpox, and he did this by infecting them with the contents of a skin lesion from a dairymaid – that is by 'vaccinating' them. During cow-pox infection the immunological system produces antibodies which are able to identify the virus, and although it takes a few days to set up production of these antibodies, they soon help to get rid of this initial (or 'primary') infection. The presence of these antibodies leads to persisting immunity to further ('secondary') infections. This works in the same way for many other virus infections, for example *Herpesvirus hominis* (see p. 124). There are some notable exceptions such as influenza, and the reason here is that the influenza virus keeps subtly changing so that antibodies made for previous infections fail to recognise the altered virus, and it is therefore able to set up what is effectively another primary infection. In the case of cow-pox, however, the primary infection not only provides immunity against a further attack of cow-pox, but also against infection by the closely related smallpox virus; the external features of these two viruses are so similar that the antibodies cannot distinguish them.

The problem with the vaccinia virus is that although the primary infection causes only a trivial lesion in normal skin, in eczematous skin it spreads like wildfire – so fast that the infection can be lethal before the protective antibodies are available. Vaccinia infection of this type, superimposed on eczema, is called 'eczema vaccinatum'. There is a very great danger of this complication occurring if a child with eczema is vaccinated against smallpox. Fortunately, smallpox vaccination is no longer obligatory and is now required only for travel to one or two exotic countries. In the event of needing to go to such a country, it is universally accepted that children with eczema are exempt from the vaccination requirement and an exemption certificate will be issued. Unfortunately, the risk remains that an eczematous child will be infected with the vaccinia virus by normal individuals who have themselves just been vaccinated. The practical message is that such persons should be regarded as a threat to any child with eczema, and physical contact between the two should be avoided. The greatest danger of all arises when other members of the child's family are vaccinated; in such circumstances, vaccination sites should be kept carefully covered until fully healed.

In sharp contrast, *all routine immunisations* may be given without any increased hazard to children with eczema, and they should therefore be given at the normal time. The widespread confusion arises at least partially from the fact that we all tend to abuse the term 'vaccination'. As I have explained, strictly speaking this means deliberate infection with vaccinia virus and is therefore not an appropriate term for immunisations against diseases other than smallpox. Vaccination in its strict sense must be avoided with children with eczema, but other immunisations are no problem.

Unfortunately, there is no satisfactory alternative to the term 'vaccine', and so we are stuck with it for all materials used for immunisation. In the past, 'vaccines' against some virus infections were made by growing the virus in hens' eggs. When the vaccine was made, it would inevitably contain a little egg protein and this could be hazardous if injected into a child with a pronounced allergy to egg. Until recently this was true of both measles and influenza vaccines, but these are both now grown in chicken cells and appear to be entirely safe, even for children highly allergic to egg. The great majority of other virus vaccines are now prepared either in human, rabbit or monkey cells. Manufacture of these vaccines also involves use of antibiotics, almost invariably neomycin. Occasionally people are allergic to neomycin, and ideally these vaccines should be avoided in such individuals. Nevertheless, it would be distinctly unusual to get a serious reaction against vaccine in such cases.

Diseases such as diphtheria, tetanus and whooping cough (pertussis) are caused by bacteria, and vaccines against them are prepared in an altogether different way. With these vaccines too there is no special risk to children with eczema.

In my view it is highly irresponsible to withhold any of the currently recommended routine immunisations from a child with eczema. Vaccination against smallpox should, on the other hand, be strictly avoided as should contact with those recently vaccinated. If you do have one of those rare children who are dangerously allergic to egg, and the child needs to have a non-routine immunisation – for example, for foreign travel – you should inquire whether the vaccine in question is grown in eggs.

10

Will My Child Get Asthma as Well?

Children with eczema are at relatively high risk of developing asthma. Like atopic eczema, asthma is a common disease and it affects 3–10% of all people at some time in their lives. Asthma similarly tends to start early in life, before the age of three years in about half of all cases. Children who already have eczema appear to have at least a three-times increased risk of developing asthma compared with other children, so somewhere between 10% and 50% of them will get asthma at some stage.

Asthma is a disorder of the tubes that take air in and out of the lungs. These tubes, or airways, have muscle in their walls that can vary their bore and therefore the ease with which air passes through. Their bore may also be reduced by swelling of their lining or by any build-up of secretions. Asthma is the result of periodic narrowing of these airways, in which all three mechanisms probably play a part. Just as in the case of eczema, there is a good deal of controversy concerning the precise cause of asthma, particularly whether it is always due to allergy. Whether or not allergy is a 'sine qua non', the end result is airways that are excessively sensitive to a wide variety of stimuli including infections, irritants, exertion and emotional stress. There are clearly close similarities with eczema. Like eczema, asthma is highly variable in severity. In many cases it is so mild that it is never recognised. In other cases it can be very disabling, and of course it can occasionally be dangerous. The best known feature of asthma is 'wheezing', a slightly musical note made mainly when breathing out and associated with shortness of breath. But wheezing occurs only when asthma is well established. A much more frequent early sign is coughing, often triggered by one of the factors I have mentioned. Coughing on exertion, or coughing in bed are particularly suspicious signs of asthma. The discovery that your child has asthma need not disconcert you too much because, as I have intimated, most cases are mild from the start and remain so. It is only in the minority that problems of any severity arise. Like eczema, asthma shows a distinct tendency to improve with time, and most children with asthma will grow out of it after a few years. It can, however, grumble on for many years and can occasionally continue into adult life, especially in some of the more severe cases. It may, like eczema, appear for the first time in adult life. Nevertheless, the most typical pattern is one of early onset and eventual complete recovery.

It is beyond the scope of this book to consider the treatment of asthma, and you should seek medical advice if you suspect that your child has asthma. If it is confirmed, however, you need not assume that this will mean more than a minor problem. Although perhaps half of all children with eczema develop asthma at some time, in very few will this ever cause serious problems.

Finally, much has been said of a 'see-saw' relationship between eczema and asthma. It is often claimed that asthma tends to appear when eczema gets better, and vice versa. I am not convinced that this is usually true. The statistics indicate clearly that eczema and asthma generally both start early in life and that both have a tendency to improve spontaneously with time. Undoubtedly some children's asthma does seem to get worse at a time when their eczema is improving, or even disappearing. Furthermore, the reverse is observed in other children. In certain cases the two certainly do seem to fluctuate in a reciprocal, see-saw fashion, and it is interesting to speculate why this should be. But in most children the two conditions seem to behave in a largely independent fashion.

11 Living with an Eczematous Child

From the very beginning, all children depend for life itself on their ability to manipulate adults in general and their parents in particular. Children who have eczema are quick to appreciate its great manipulative value, and rarely hesitate to make full use of this. Such children soon realise that their eczema can be used to secure special treatment, so long as a failure to secure it is marked by a tantrum disguised as a fearsome bout of scratching – if possible ending in the drawing of blood. Children will do this quite naturally, instinctively and subconsciously – at least initially. If it is successful, this manipulation may later on become conscious, and this is when it becomes undesirable and hazardous to the child's development as a normal member of society. What can be done about this? Being aware of the problem is half the battle. Do not let the pattern of events develop in which a bout of scratching will always end up with your child getting exactly what he or she wants. Temper tantrums which take the form of scratching have to be ignored just like any other kind. Once your child realises that this sort of thing won't work, he or she will stop doing it.

Children with eczema need never be scarred by the disease itself, either physically or mentally. They may, however, suffer lasting harm as a result of having been treated as 'different' from other children, even though this may have been done with the best possible motives. It is vital to treat your eczematous child no differently from the way you would treat any other child. The emotional effect of severe eczema on a child is not the same as it would be on an adult. Small children live from day to day, even from minute to minute. Fortunately, they rarely have the foresight to become disheartened and quickly recover from bad periods. However dreadful their eczema has been, they quickly forget. The great majority will eventually recover physically, but it is to a great extent up to you to make sure that when this happens they will be no different from other people. Most important of all is not to be overprotective. Let your child do everything that other children do, even if it does make the skin a little worse. You can of course try to interest them preferentially in things that do not make their eczema worse, but if they desperately want to ride horses or go swimming – activities which can have an aggravating effect – don't stop them. Don't ask if they can be excused PE or games at school, and don't stop them going to birthday parties because they are on special diets. A single afternoon's deviation from a diet is unlikely to do as much harm in the long term as stopping them joining in the fun. This is the point, not to pay for short-term gains by long-term losses.

Tension often builds up in families where a child has eczema. We have already considered the tension that can be generated by the child's attempts, conscious or subconscious, to get his own way. Your other children will resent any additional attention given to a brother or sister with eczema, and this is another reason why you must make quite sure you are not manipulated. Some extra attention is unavoidable, because it takes time to give the treatment and special diets may mean special food. It is important, however, to be aware of the jealousies that such 'special' treatment may arouse. If you are careful to compensate for it, it need never become a problem. Husbands and wives may envy the attention given to an eczematous child, in just the same way. Arguments about the child's treatment are common, and are often symptomatic of this kind of resentment. Such arguments are liable in their turn to provoke unnecessary additional anxiety in the child. Occasionally, such disagreements are actually capitalized on by a manipulative child. It is very important indeed never to let your child become aware of the worry you feel over his skin disease. Try hard not to allow yourself to be more distressed by your child's problem than the child is himself. I am sure this happens more easily than one might think.

People outside the family constitute another potential source of tension. Because eczema is both common and visible, everyone reserves the right to know best. There are literally hundreds of theories about the cause of the disease, and just as many miraculous 'cures'. The worst kind of reaction from an outsider is the inhuman one of withdrawal, in which your child is regarded as a threat, unclean or infectious. This is one problem that parents almost always encounter, sooner or later. Do your best not to be upset by it. Whenever the opportunity arises, strike a blow for eczema sufferers everywhere by gently explaining that eczema is not the result of lack of hygiene, nor is it contagious. Don't hide your child away; more good is done by letting people get used to the idea that he or she has eczema. Being hidden away can also have a bad effect on the child, who is unlikely ever to become ashamed of his condition unless others teach him to be. When people offer their theories, listen politely. If you don't want them to, try to avoid eczema as a subject of conversation and especially try not to appear desperate. If you complain to others about doctors, you give them carte blanche!

I am often asked by parents what they should do about their child scratching, and this really is a tricky problem. Parents' distress at seeing their child tearing himself to pieces naturally leads them to try to intervene. Unfortunately, this intervention may seriously aggravate matters. Never shout at your child to stop doing what is partly an involuntary reaction to the intense itching. Whereas scratching often relieves other forms of irritation in the skin, in eczema it seems only to make it worse until it is substituted by pain and this will not happen until serious damage has been done. If you do shout, you will only heighten the tension and further intensify the irritation. Your child will interpret the shouting as a sign that you do not love him or her. The same is true of any physical attempt to prevent scratching. Never punish a child for scratching. But having said what you shouldn't do, what should you do? All you really can do is to make every effort, firstly to distract the child's attention away from his skin and, secondly, to reduce the amount of damage actually done as a result of the scratching. Distracting the child is more difficult than screaming at him, and more time-consuming, but it is the right way. Try going out or playing with your child; do anything that will focus attention on something other than the skin. If simple distractions fail, pop the child in a bath; this can often provide surprisingly effective relief. An alternative is to apply generous quantities of a moisturiser such as Unguentum Merck, Ultrabase, Boots E45 Cream or Aqueous Cream. This will at least provide a layer of protective lubrication to reduce the damage done by any scratching. If all this fails to relieve the irritation you should let your child scratch but with the least possible destructive effect. Make sure always that his nails are as short as possible and free of jagged edges. Daily attention with the nail-file is the best approach. Encourage your child to apply a moisturiser while scratching. Try to promote rubbing rather than scratching. It is sometimes a good idea to do the rubbing or scratching yourself, but gently.

12 What About Education?

It has often been suggested that children with eczema are of above-average intelligence. Careful studies have shown that this is a myth, however, and that in terms of intelligence children with eczema are indistinguishable from normal children. Intelligence is a measure of potential and, in a sense, what is more important is actual achievement – do eczematous children actually do as well academically as their normal counterparts? The answer to this is that overall they almost certainly do not. Their educational progress is hampered in a number of ways. The most obvious is their frequently irregular attendance at school. In addition, they are likely to find it difficult to maintain concentration in the face of any degree of skin irritation. Attentiveness can also be impaired by the soporific effect of antihistamines (see p. 83). I have the feeling that some parents actually try to shield their eczematous children from the academic pressures of school, in the belief that these pressures represent an unfair additional burden on them. But, as I suggested in the last chapter, any action that tends to isolate children with eczema is in fact only likely to make matters worse. As in all other facets of your child's life, in educational matters it is important to try to provide an environment that is as normal as possible.

The education problem is, of course, more or less restricted to children with more severe eczema; the worse the eczema, the greater the potential problem. Paradoxically, education is of particular importance to those with severe eczema, because a wide variety of possible careers are going to be unsuitable for them. Any job which involves contact of the skin with irritants is best avoided, and this limitation should be borne in mind throughout the child's education. Every year I see student nurses who had eczema when they were children. The eczema later cleared up, as it tends to, but the constant exposure to antiseptics and detergents that is an inevitable part of the job is likely to provoke a recurrence; often this will mean that nursing has to be given up altogether. It would have been better if this danger had been foreseen and a more suitable career planned at an earlier stage.

Similarly unsuitable jobs for girls include hairdressing and cooking. These are jobs which are likely to provoke renewed eczema long after it has cleared up and will certainly flare up eczema which is already active. Any job in which a perfect skin is essential is clearly going to be a dodgy proposition for any girl with eczema. Though I have met a number of successful models who have eczema, for obvious reasons this is a profession best avoided. Where the hands are on show, hand eczema may cause real problems. Almost any job in catering, for example, is likely to be barred to those with hand eczema.

For boys, almost any kind of manual work is likely to make matters worse. Obviously unsuitable jobs are those of mechanic, carpenter, bricklayer or painter. The safest are the more clerical types of job, and generally those which require the brains rather than the hands. This is exactly why a good education is really more important for those with eczema than for those without.

I want to outline a few principles that I believe may help in the successful education of eczematous children, though they will not all be appropriate in every case. I hope that any education professional reading this book will forgive any naivety on my part, and I imagine they would not agree with all I say. I feel that there is often much to be gained from eczematous children starting school a little early, wherever possible. Firstly, this may help to give them a headstart to compensate for absences that may occur later. Secondly, I think they often benefit from the social experience of school, and from the periodic physical separation from their mothers that school entails. This can provide the basis for a less intense and more independent relationship between mother and child, something which is generally beneficial. The greater activity that goes with school turns the child's attention outwards, helping to prevent development of the introverted personality that so often goes with eczema.

When your child is about to start at school, it is a good idea to speak to his or her prospective teacher. Tell the teacher that your child has eczema, and explain the kinds of treatment being used. If the teacher knows little about eczema, a little general information may be welcomed, and you should particularly lay emphasis on the fact that the disease is not contagious. Other parents may later ask the teacher what is wrong with your child and it helps if clear answers can be given them from the start. Make sure to have a word with the school nurse when there is one. Ask her if she would be prepared to apply creams and ointments if necessary. If she will do this, it is a good plan to provide her with a supply of whatever moisturiser you prefer. This helps her by giving her something she can do for your child when and if the need arises. If your child is on any special form of diet, it is obviously important to check that the school can cope with this. If not, you may need to provide packed lunches and in special circumstances you may even need to take him or her for lunch.

As often as you can, take the opportunity to tell other children's parents what is wrong with your child, as this will help to prevent them being told to keep away. If you discover that he is being taunted because of his skin, let the teacher know and, if possible, the parents of the responsible child (this may call for considerable tact). It is an important part of the education of normal children that they come to terms with those less fortunate than themselves. If your child seems depressed, ask if he has been teased about his skin – this can help by bringing the problem into the open.

Sometimes it is suggested to parents that their eczematous child might do better at some type or other of special school. It seems to me that such recommendations often reflect the inadequacies of the school and its staff rather than any real need for change of school from the child's point of view. As in all aspects of your child's life, as normal as possible an approach is best. If you want help with this kind of problem do not hesitate to approach your doctor and suggest that you discuss the situation with a social worker. Sometimes a change of school is a good idea, but this is the exception. I have, on the other hand, known two particularly severely eczematous childen whose lives have been revolutionised by going away to boarding schools, with their more outdoor and self-reliant emphasis.

The physical education side of school activity can be a special problem. Your child may find undressing embarrassing, and this requires sympathy on everybody's part. Hard physical exertion can lead to quite marked irritation of the skin and, where there is a choice, activities that lead to the least irritation should obviously be preferred. Nevertheless, as far as possible eczematous children should take part in physical education and games to avoid being different, even if a degree of aggravation of their eczema is the price for this. Do think hard before suggesting that your child be exempted altogether from sports.

Absences from school can become a problem. You should avoid keeping your child away from school, firstly because of the fact once again that it makes him different. Very occasionally, frequent absences are inevitable and he will then need extra help. This is something for you to discuss with your child's teacher. We have been able to arrange home tutoring for one or two children who have fallen behind, and in every case that I recall, this has been a great success, allowing the child to catch up and re-enter the normal educational system in due course.

In summary, do all you can to get your child as good an education as possible. The emphasis should be on normal treatment at school, and your main task is quietly to try to prevent problems before they arise by talking to teachers, school nurses and other parents. I am constantly heartened by how well severely eczematous children can do in spite of all their problems. Understanding on the part of the teachers and fellow pupils will help them immeasurably.

13 Will My Next Child Get Eczema?

Parents of children with severe eczema often ask me if any further children they may have will also be affected. Some parents feel that if the risk were high they would prefer not to take it. In an earlier chapter, we briefly considered the way eczema is inherited (p. 12). In fact, the situation seems to be a very complicated one, and it would be worth while looking at it a little more closely. Maybe I should start by discussing how characteristics are passed on from one generation to the next.

Physical differences between people, say the colour of their eyes, result from slight differences in the structure of specific proteins. Proteins consist of chains of subunits known as amino-acids. There are about 20 different amino-acids which can be arranged in an almost infinite variety of sequences, just as the 26 letters of the alphabet can be used to make thousands of different words. The body is able to make up proteins very precisely because it carries a set of exact plans in each and every one of its cells. These plans are called 'genes', and for each and every protein there is a corresponding gene. The genes are arranged in strings known as 'chromosomes'. Each person gets his first complete set of genes from his parents, half a set from one parent and half a set from the other.

Some diseases are inherited in a precise way. A good example is achondroplasia. Achondroplasics are familiar to most people as circus dwarfs, a job for which they are physically particularly well suited. Achondroplasics have a defect in the growth of their bones that causes dwarfing, though they are in all other ways perfectly healthy. If an achondroplasic marries a normal person, half the resulting children will be achondroplasics, the other half will be normal. This is because a child gets half his genes from each parent, so each child has a 50:50 chance of inheriting the achondroplasic gene. This is an example of the simplest pattern of inheritance. Other conditions are passed on in a more complex way. In some, the children will have a one-in-four chance of inheriting the condition; in others, half the boys will inherit it but none of the girls, and so on. Many conditions depend on inheriting combinations of genes; this is known as 'polygenic' inheritance. In polygenic conditions, the influence of the environment may be very strong, making matters even more complicated. Height is a good example of a characteristic inherited in this way. Height is highly variable, not merely something you have or don't have. A large number of genes determine the potential height of an individual, but environmental factors, particularly nutrition, will actually decide whether the potential height is reached. The height of one's parents is important, and the potential height of children is approximately half-way between the heights of their parents. If one's parents are tall, one will almost certainly be tall; if one's parents are short one should expect to be short – unless, of course, one's parents are short because of poor nutrition rather than their genes.

The pattern of inheritance of eczema is very similar to the inheritance of height. One inherits the potential to develop eczema, not eczema itself (Fig 13.1). Environmental factors decide whether one actually develops it or not. How bad it is probably also results from a combination of inheritance and environment. If it is true, as we suspect, that between 10% and 15% of all children develop a degree of atopic eczema at some time, then we should perhaps consider it more as a variant of normal than as a disease. It is, of course, only a small proportion of these children in whom it represents a real problem, just as it is only in a very small proportion of children that shortness is a real problem.

One's risk of developing eczema can be related, albeit somewhat imprecisely, to the presence or absence of atopic diseases in one's parents – that is, atopic eczema, asthma or hayfever. If *one* parent has or has had one of these conditions, the child's risk of developing atopic eczema will be about double that of a child whose parents have never had any of these. If *both* parents have or have had any atopic disease, the risk of eczema in their

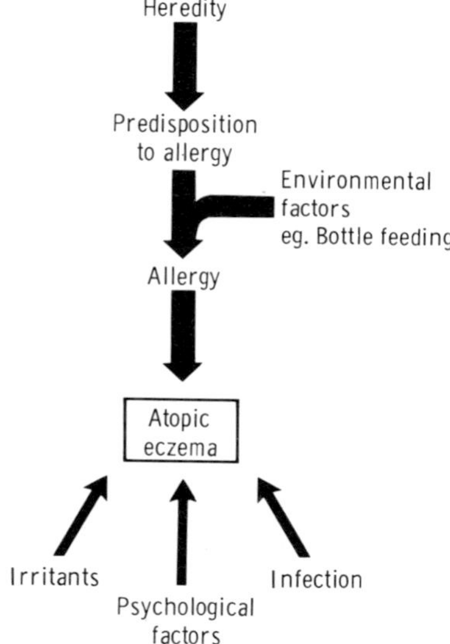

Fig. 13.1

child is doubled again. In a study done a few years ago in Sweden, atopic eczema was reported by parents to have occurred in 8% of all children by the age of seven years. Where there was no history at all of parental atopic disease, the figure was 6%; where one parent had such a history it was 12%; where both did, the figure reached 33%. But what if neither parent has a history of atopic disease, but a brother or sister does? In fact, having such a brother or sister increases the risk to about the same degree as having a parent with atopic disease does – to about double. Having a brother or sister *as well as* one parent with atopic disease does not appear to increase the risk any further. Figures are not available showing the position if a child has two or more brothers or sisters with atopic disease, but one would imagine that having two or more affected brothers or sisters would be very much like having two affected parents.

If parents, or brothers or sisters, have a history of eczema itself, rather than just asthma or hayfever, then the risk is increased even further. This implies that in addition to genes transmitting risk of atopic disease in general there are others which transmit the risk of eczema in particular (Fig. 13.2).

What all this means is that if you already have a child with eczema, your next will have about a one-in-four chance of developing eczema. I suspect that many parents worry that the risk may be higher and will find it reassuring that the actual risk is much less than 50:50. What they should also bear in mind is that atopic eczema is usually a fairly mild disease, so that even if their next child is affected the odds are that the condition will be less severe – another reason to feel reassured.

	Overall risk for whole population	No history of atopic disease in family	One parent and/or one brother/sister			Two parents and/or two brothers/sisters		
			any atopic disease	asthma/hayfever	eczema	any atopic disease	asthma/hayfever	eczema
Risk of developing atopic eczema	10%	5%	20%	15%	25%	40%	30%	50%

Fig. 13.2 Table showing the statistical risk of a child developing eczema, and the increased risk if one or two first-degree relatives (i.e. brothers, sisters or parents) themselves have atopic disorders. It can be seen that the risk is highest where relatives have or have had atopic eczema rather than asthma or hayfever.

Can we do anything to Reduce the Risk?

Parents who are worried about having a child with eczema often ask if there is anything they can do to reduce the risk. The hereditary part of the risk they obviously cannot change, but it seems likely that the environmental contribution could be modified. For example, there is evidence that risk of eczema depends to some extent on month of birth, those children born during the autumn being at increased risk, and it has been suggested that this increased risk may reflect the relatively heavier exposure to house dust mite which occurs at this time of year. Whatever the real explanation, it seems that events occurring during the first few weeks of life are crucial in determining the likelihood of an at-risk infant actually developing eczema.

One of the most important factors appears to be the way an infant is fed. There is now increasingly reliable evidence that exclusively breastfed infants have a reduced risk of atopic eczema, though it is still unclear whether this reflects a protective effect of breastmilk or a harmful effect of the usual cow's milk-based bottlefeeds. Recent studies suggest that feeding nothing other than breastmilk for the first three months of life may reduce the likelihood of eczema to a half or a third of what it would be if the infant were bottlefed. Exclusive breastfeeding means no supplementary bottlefeeds at all. Unfortunately, it remains common practice in maternity wards to bottlefeed newly-born infants at night in order not to disturb the mother. If a baby is delivered by forceps or by caesarean section it will often be taken away from its mother for the first 24 hours, during which time it will be bottlefed. I am glad to say that things are changing in these respects. Not only is it best for the baby to be breastfed from the outset, but this removal of demand for milk from the breast may actually spoil a mother's chance of every establishing an adequate supply of milk. I would urge any mother to plan to breastfeed her baby, but particularly where there is any family history of atopic disease. Talk to your family doctor, obstetrician and midwife before the baby is born. Make it clear that breastfeeding is your firm intention, and that you do not wish supplements other than water – which should be given in the form of dextrose – to be given to your baby without your express permission. *Breast is Best* by Drs Penny and Andrew Stanway (Pan Books Ltd) provides an excellent introduction to breastfeeding, and I strongly recommend reading it at some time during pregnancy.

But what can you do should breastfeeding be impossible for one reason or another? This is a difficult one. There is some evidence that a soya milk is preferable to a cow's milk-based infant feed in terms of increased risk of eczema, but the difference is probably not a great one. There are now several soya feeds on the market that are suitable for infants: they include Prosobee (Mead Johnson), Velactin (Wander), Wysoy (Wyeth) and Formula S (Cow & Gate). A unique infant feed has recently become available. Called Pregestimil, it is made from casein, a protein obtained from cow's milk. During the manufacturing process this protein is 'hydrolysed' – that is, broken down to very short chains of amino-acids. This process removes the protein's ability to cause allergy and the feed is theoretically non-antigenic. This should make it an ideal alternative to breast milk where one is needed, but there are two snags. The first is the very high cost. The second is that the suitability of this feed for small babies is not yet 100% established. It should not be used, therefore unless the risk is a high one and your family doctor, obstetrician or paediatrician is prepared to prescribe it.

If possible, you should aim at feeding your baby nothing other than your own milk for the first four months of its life. The protective effect may be even greater if you continue breast feeding for longer than this, though you should be aware that human milk alone is not a nutritionally adequate diet for babies older than six months.

While exclusive breast feeding does reduce the risk of eczema, it does not eliminate it altogether, and many breast fed babies get eczema. There are probably at least three reasons why this happens.

The first is the difficulty of ensuring that breastfeeding is truly exclusive. I have already drawn attention to the still all-too-common practice in hospitals of giving babies surreptitious bottlefeeds during their first hours of life. This practice is well-meant, but ill-advised, and it may entirely nullify the benefits of subsequent exclusive breastfeeding.

The second reason is that babies are exposed to antigens other than those in their food. They come into contact with airborne antigens just the same as everyone else – that is, pollen spores, animal dander and, above all, house dust mites. As I mentioned, there is evidence that babies born in the autumn, when house dust mites are most populous, may be more likely to develop eczema than babies born at any other season. For this reason, it would seem wise to make an effort to reduce the population of house dust mites in the immediate environment of an at-risk baby (see p. 101). Clearly, there is no place for a dog or cat in a family with an at-risk baby.

The third reason is that food antigens from the mother's own diet may be transmitted, albeit in minute amounts, to her baby in her own milk. It may seem incredible, but there is no doubt that this does occur. After a lactating mother drinks cow's milk, intact cow's milk proteins may be discovered in her milk. That this could provoke allergy is demonstrated by the fact that some exclusively breastfed babies develop antibodies to these cow's milk proteins before a drop of actual cow's milk has crossed their lips. Although such antigens are present in breast milk in quantities sufficient to induce an allergic sensitisation, they are rarely present in the amounts required to provoke full-blown allergic reactions. Although some babies do appear to develop eczema as a reaction to food allergens while still exclusively breastfed, it is more characteristic for the eczema to appear first on weaning. It is very common indeed for babies to develop their eczema within one or two days of having their first cow's milk feeds. This is much too quick for the allergy to have been induced by these first feeds, and it implies that such babies are already sensitive.

It is therefore a logical question whether breastfeeding mothers should eliminate cow's milk, and possibly certain other foods, from their own diet. Although the principle is soundly based, the best way to put it into practice is not established, since no-one actually knows for certain which foods should be avoided, when this avoidance should start or how strict it must be. I can only give my own personal views on the subject.

First of all, I do not think that any mother-to-be should contemplate eliminating foods from her diet while breastfeeding unless her child is at high risk of developing eczema. The higher the risk, the more worth while such a manoeuvre is likely to be. I feel that it is only in relation to eggs and cow's milk that a strong case can be made out for avoidance. If eggs and cow's milk are avoided, adequately nutritious alternatives must be incorporated into the diet in compensation. This means both an alternative source of first-class protein and calcium, which are probably best supplied in the form of extra meat and calcium tablets. If extra calcium is not taken, it will be extracted from the mother's bones and teeth to maintain the supply in her milk for as long as possible, a process which clearly poses a threat to her long-term health. Probably the ideal form in which to take supplementary calcium is as a single effervescent Sandocal tablet daily. Ideally, this regimen should be started a few days before delivery, and continued throughout lactation. In order to succeed in avoiding egg and cow's milk protein completely, advice would be needed from a dietitian. However, I doubt whether it is necessary for the avoidance to be obsessional for it to be beneficial, and I imagine that the very small amounts of these proteins found – for example, in biscuits and cake – would be more or less irrelevant.

On various occasions I have been asked if similar precautions should also be taken during pregnancy. There is increasing evidence that some babies are already sensitised to foods, particularly eggs and cow's milk, at birth, implying that food antigens can cross the placenta intact. An attempt to reduce one's intake of these items, at least during the last six months of pregnancy, therefore makes no less sense than doing so during lactation. Perhaps much of the harm done during pregnancy and lactation results from the constant heavy pressure to which women are subjected at these times to consume eggs and milk in truly massive quantities. Such advice appears ill-founded in the case of mothers of potentially allergic infants.

Now we come to the problem of weaning the at-risk baby from exclusive breastfeeding. Introduction of some solids should ideally be instituted no earlier than the fourth month and no later than the seventh. The fifth month is probably the ideal time. Our present state of knowledge does not allow very precise advice to be given, but in my view it is wise to avoid giving an at-risk baby any cow's milk until the age of at least one year, and egg protein until at least two years. Cow's milk avoidance implies avoidance of all foods containing cow's milk protein, which means keeping a careful eye on the contents of prepared baby foods. Any foods containing whey or casein should therefore not be used.

You should aim at breastfeeding after each solid feed until the end of this first year. If you can not do this, a soya milk may be the best alternative and there is little to choose from the four excellent preparations mentioned earlier.

Introduce vegetables and fruits first of all. Suitable vegetables include lentils, peas or beans, cabbage, broccoli, Brussels sprouts, cauliflower, carrots, swedes or turnips. These should be boiled carefully because overcooking destroys much of their nutritional value, and then sieved or mashed. A little milk-free margarine – for example, Tomor – may be added for its softening effect. Potato should be preferred to cereal at this stage as a source of carbohydrate. It is a good idea to mix boiled mashed potato with other vegetables. Suitable fruits include mashed banana, stewed apple or pear, or mashed tinned fruits such as peaches or apricots. Give such feeds three times daily, finishing off with a breastfeed.

Introduce some minced meat after a month. Turkey and lamb are a good choice as there is no overlap of proteins with egg and cow's milk, though in practice there is little risk with chicken and beef. Serve with vegetables and potato.

After another month, introduce cereals. Rice is a good one to start with. At this stage you could also try fish, which should initially be white fish such as haddock or cod.

Clearly, there is for the present no way of guaranteeing prevention of eczema by the kinds of maneouvres we have been discussing. In the light of our current knowledge, these precautions nevertheless seem sensible, and no doubt they do lead to some reduction in the risk. It is in this area of prevention that some of our greatest hopes for the future now lie.

Appendix
The National Eczema Society

If your child has eczema or if you have eczema yourself, much can be gained through contact with other parents and sufferers. A few years ago, some patients, parents and doctors got together and formed a society, which they called the National Eczema Society, whose object was to help sufferers, and those who care for them, to help themselves. The society attempts to achieve this in several ways. Firstly, it provides opportunities for people with eczematous children or spouses, or with eczema themselves, to meet. Great comfort can come through sharing experiences and the feeling of no longer being alone. A society of this type can also help by making the problem of eczema better known to people generally, perhaps making it less mysterious, less threatening and less misunderstood. A more sympathetic attitude in people at large would help enormously. Not least among the aims of the society are those of improving the treatment and understanding of eczema; these are accomplished by interesting both doctors and scientists in the problem of eczema, and by financing specific research projects.

The National Eczema Society also publishes a magazine called *Exchange* four times a year; this carries articles by doctors and other health professionals and also provides an exchange of information between members. Regular meetings provide the opportunity to hear professionals talk in a 'down to earth' way (one hopes!) about eczema and the problems it causes, and interesting discussion often follows. The society has an office which is staffed during working hours, and from which information of all sorts can be obtained, at:

Tavistock House North
Tavistock Square
London WC1 9SR
Telephone: 01 – 388 4097

Index